Praise for *So*

'A brave, vital and necessary b

'This is a great book, and an important one. It's the one I would give to any friend who I observed struggling with those issues, as it's written in a genuinely human way, devoid of psychobabble, moralizing, victimhood embracing and judgement. It comes from a place of hard-won experience, told with total honesty. It will do more than just save lives, it will help those saved lives feel like they're genuinely worth living'

Irvine Welsh

'An honest, funny account of how we're all capable of changing for the better'

Seth Meyers

'This book tells it like it is in an honest and down to earth way that men who find it hard to talk about mental health will be able to relate to easily. Sam really knows his stuff on this subject and is very frank about his struggles. A great, motivating book that can really help – every bloke should read it'

Shaun Ryder

'A funny, wise and above all valuable book. An arm around your shoulder from your next best friend'

Danny Wallace

'Finally, a book on mental health that strikes the right note'

Reaction

Sam Delaney is a journalist and broadcaster whose work has featured in the *Guardian*, *Telegraph* and talkSPORT. He is former editor of *Heat* magazine. Sam also co-hosts the popular podcast *Top Flight Time Machine*. Since 2020 he has hosted *The Reset*, a podcast about men and mental health. He is the author of three previous books.

Sort Your Head Out

Mental health without all the bollocks

Sam Delaney

CONSTABLE

CONSTABLE

First published in Great Britain in 2023 by Constable
This paperback edition published in 2024 by Constable

1 3 5 7 9 10 8 6 4 2

Copyright © Sam Delaney, 2023

A CIP catalogue record for this book
is available from the British Library.

ISBN: 978-1-40871-709-7

Typeset in Minion Pro by SX Composing DTP, Rayleigh, Essex
Printed and bound in Great Britain by Clays Ltd, Elcograf, S.p.A.

Papers used by Constable are from well-managed forests
and other responsible sources.

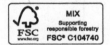

MIX
Supporting
responsible forestry
FSC® C104740

Constable
An imprint of
Little, Brown Book Group
Carmelite House
50 Victoria Embankment
London EC4Y 0DZ

An Hachette UK Company

www.hachette.co.uk

www.littlebrown.co.uk

To Theo, Dom and Cas

Contents

PART 2: SOBER

Introduction

Alexandra Palace, December 2014. It was that period between Christmas and New Year during which I, like many others, am particularly prone to bouts of misery. But this year I had a plan to stave off the Black Dog. I'd booked tickets to see the darts with my eldest brother Theo and my nineteen-year-old nephew, Fred. Christmas darts seemed like the most fun thing in the world: a building full of lads in fancy dress, getting wasted, singing daft songs, watching professional sportsmen throw things with implausible accuracy. How could anyone feel sad at a place like that?

When we got there I was already pretty hammered, having fuelled up in various pubs along the way. There was a very wide, very deep, very boisterous queue of people outside. When I finally got to the front, I was surprised by the extent of the security measures: metal detectors like at the airport and a squad of moody bouncers pushing and shoving everyone around. The atmosphere felt a bit volatile. 'This is brilliant!' I said to my brother.

But it didn't stay brilliant for long. One of the bouncers began to subject me to an aggressive pat down which included a rummage through my pockets. 'What the fuck are you doing?!' I asked. He ignored me and slipped his fingers into the little money pocket of my jeans as if he knew what he was going to find there. Yes, it was an unimaginative place to keep my cocaine but, in fairness, I had not expected such a thorough body search.

He found both wraps immediately, slipped them out and held them up to my face to demonstrate his discovery. 'Right you, wait here,' he said and motioned for some of his colleagues to come over and get involved. Before I knew it, one of them had hold of my arms from behind. What the hell was happening?

'OK, fine, you found my drugs, well done,' I said. 'Bit of an affront to my personal space and human rights to be honest, but I'm not one to make a fuss so just keep hold of them and let me in so I can carry on drinking.'

Like I say, I was wasted. And the bouncers weren't playing ball. It quickly became apparent that not only was I going to be denied entry but that they were planning to impose further punishment. They muttered into their walkie-talkies while eying me contemptuously and I became convinced that they were summoning the police to arrest me on drug charges.

So I did what any other wired, pissed-up idiot who'd been captured by security guards at the darts would do. I wrestled myself free of their clutches, began to flail my arms around like a crazy person, shouted 'FUCK OFF!' at no one in particular and just charged for the exit door, shoving a number of innocent bystanders aside in the process. I was outside in the forecourt before security knew what was happening, shouting back at them, 'I AM OUT OF YOUR JURISDICTION NOW, CUNTS!'

I could – and maybe should – have just cut my losses and gone home at that point. But instead, I walked round the other side of the building and negotiated with someone at the VIP entrance to let me into the venue for £200 in cash, which I had withdrawn on a credit card because I had no real money left in my bank account. Pleased with my defiance of the venue's uptight security policies, I waltzed into the thrilling mayhem of the main darts arena. My brother and nephew, having assumed they wouldn't be seeing me again for the rest of the night, were quite surprised to witness me charging towards them, wild-eyed and mad for it, bellowing, 'Stand up if you love the darts!' with a pint of lager in each hand.

Nobody could stop me having my fun. Nobody. But was I happy? It was hard to tell at this stage.

Next, I noticed a Sky TV crew walking through the crowd, picking out eye-catching members of the crowd to capture on camera. *I'll have some of that!* I thought to myself, brimming with drunken hubris. I picked up a large sheet of paper that had been distributed by one of the bookmakers for spectators to write messages on. I grabbed a pen and quickly wrote 'Marry me Anna!' then rushed towards the cameraman, who was only too happy to film my stupid romantic gesture for the entertainment of the viewers at home.

Back in the leafy suburbs of south-west London, the Anna in question had just put our two small children to bed and tuned in to see if she could catch a quick glimpse of me on the telly. She was confronted by the spectacle of me, her husband of nine years, bloated and mad, clearly drunk and with traces of white powder caked around his nostrils, inexplicably proposing to her on a crumpled sheet of paper on national TV. Anna was not touched by this gesture. Anna was confused, annoyed and deeply concerned.

The kids were three and seven years old at the time. I should have probably been at home, watching a box set with my wife and having a herbal tea in my slippers. That's perhaps how I had envisaged life turning out by the time I was thirty-nine. It had always seemed like it was heading that way. I'd had some fun in my time. I'd done the big nights out and the weekend drug-dabbling in my teens and twenties. But by my thirties I had a successful career, my own house, a lovely wife and two incredible kids. I was respectable. I had everything I had ever wanted. My whole life seemed to be on track. Until it wasn't.

I wonder how other people saw me that night? I doubt most of the other lads at the darts would have noticed anything exceptional about my behaviour. I mean, Christmas darts at Alexandra Palace is widely known to be pretty raucous – I felt as if you'd need to do something truly extraordinary to stand out as particularly problematic. I'd heard that, the night before, someone had puked in a pint glass up on the balcony, then tipped it on to the heads of the people standing below. That's where the bar was set, bad behaviour-wise. By comparison, some dickhead getting caught with a bit of gear then proposing to a woman he was already married to on TV was really quite vanilla.

My brother certainly noticed that I was acting slightly out of character. I remember him looking at me as I re-entered the arena with the concerned eye of a radiologist who'd just spotted a slightly unusual shadow on a chest X-ray. He knew I'd always been one of the lads but, suddenly, I was acting up in a rather more outlandish manner than usual. My nephew, who might once have respected and admired me as an uncle who was wise, fun and capable, was probably seeing me now as the fat, pissed-up knobhead I had become.

As for Anna, sitting at home watching me on Sky, she would have simply seen me as a great disappointment. She was right to. I was failing her and I was failing myself. Deep down, I knew this and was just waiting for a great reckoning, a rock bottom or a grand ultimatum to put a halt to my antics. Frustratingly, it just never seemed to arrive. How was I getting away with this shit night after night?

While that question bubbled menacingly in a corner of my subconscious, the more suggestible part of my brain told a quite different story. It told me that I was, in fact, an absolute legend. Swept up in the boozy excitement of the evening, I thought I was a real hero, living free of society's stuffy conventions and giving the middle finger to the authorities who tried to stand between me and a good time. That was how I felt for a couple of hours, at least.

But later that night, as I lay in bed beside Anna, yet again trying and failing to get to sleep, the familiar feelings of shame, guilt, paranoia and self-hatred engulfed me.

What came first, the addictions or the sadness? That's an easy one: it was definitely the sadness.

I'd always felt a bit uncomfortable with myself and struggled to be alone with my own thoughts. At an early age I'd realised that drink and drugs were a pretty reliable way of numbing all those shitty feelings. I hadn't always been an addict, but I had always been an addict waiting to happen. I had never learned how to cope with uncomfortable feelings other than to distract myself from them. Over the years, I had used all sorts of things as distractions: work, food, shopping, exercise – anything that diverted my attention away from deeper, more difficult thoughts and emotions and gave me a quick dose of joy, however fleeting and synthetic. Drugs and booze were just the same as all the other distractions. Only they were better, faster acting and more reliable. There was always a chance I would come to rely on them too heavily.

It was strange that this had started to happen in my mid-thirties when I thought all of the big risks of earlier adulthood had been averted. Your twenties can be a rough time, with the uncertainties that surround relationships and career. I'd got through that period relatively unscathed. I figured if I hadn't become an addict by now, then I never would. But like Mafia hitmen, my demons came and got me when I least expected.

I had always been a Jack the Lad. I grew up as the youngest of four brothers. Beer, football and piss-taking defined the dynamics of our household. We fought and shouted and got drunk. As the youngest by a seven-year margin, I was often on the sharp end of the bullying. So I had learned to hold my own – first in the banter, then in the hedonism – from an early age.

The laddish persona is often portrayed as inherently toxic but, I can't lie, it's also a right laugh. Plus, the idea that everyone who likes beer and football is also a moronic bigot is a myth perpetuated by snobs. Yes, I went to a comprehensive school, grew up in a council house and have a season ticket at West Ham. But I also went to university and read the *Guardian*. For most of my childhood my mum was a secretary at a building firm and we often relied on benefits to make ends meet. My dad, who didn't live with us, was a successful advertising executive who took us to nice restaurants at weekends. People can mix and match all of those conflicting elements of my background as they wish. I do it myself. Your sense of identity has a big role to play in your mental health. Your perspective on who you are, how you should act and where you should be in life steers your sense of self-worth. My perspective on this stuff has often veered about wildly, as you will see as this story unfolds. But one thing that I have always consistently enjoyed is being one of the lads. Not only because it is fun but also because it is comforting. There is a simplicity to the worldview that I can really get behind.

There are toxic interpretations of the term 'lad' that might suggest antisocial behaviour, intolerance and boorish idiocy. It all comes down to semantics, but I'd call those sort of men not 'lads' but 'wankers'. To me, being a lad is not about being a hooligan. It's about excitement, irreverence and camaraderie. It has brought me good times and beautiful friendships; it has also been another form of protection from the darker feelings that permanently floated in the back of my mind. For most of my life I took nothing seriously, least of all myself.

By the way, I haven't had a bad life and my childhood was pretty happy. I wasn't a victim of abuse; I hadn't suffered any sudden bereavements or been separated from loved ones at an early age. I've not been held back by prejudice. For the most part, my life has been fortunate and full of love. This was another reason why I forbade myself from ever dwelling on my mental health. I thought any feelings of sadness and discomfort were daft and unwarranted; to give them the time of day would be a pathetic indulgence. Feeling sorry for yourself was for hippies, whingers and spoiled brats. I wouldn't allow myself to acknowledge my own pain. But, like any other human that ever lived – irrespective of the background they came from or the circumstances of their existence – I felt pain. Comparing and contrasting my pain to that of other, less fortunate, people was a technique I used to try and snap myself out of glumness. But it was a shit technique because it only served to compound all that pain with feelings of shame. It did nothing to help dig the pain out by the roots.

To do that, I needed to confront my sadness and anxiety at its source. To identify the stuff that might have made me feel shit about myself and resentful of others; and to try and work out a way past those feelings. That was never going to be possible while I was constantly off my face.

The combined pressures of parenting and career had left me exhausted and miserable by the time I was in my late thirties. I had been trying way too hard to be a perfect family man and a model professional, and I had wound up being neither. I was overstretched and overwhelmed and had sunk into bad habits in a misguided attempt to hold it all together. My marriage was in peril. My career teetered on the edge of disaster. I was in a state of constant financial panic. Each of these problems fed off each other. I was in a cycle of inebriation, worry and conflict.

Shitfaced nights at the darts weren't the half of it. The uglier and more worrying side was the stuff I did out of plain sight: the all-day solo binges in the corner of the local pub; the late nights getting wasted in the front room while my wife and kids were asleep upstairs; the empty vodka bottles hidden in the filing cabinet; the nights where I would lie in darkness beside my sleeping wife, wide awake and sweating – fighting back tears of panic and misery. Urgh.

Drink and drugs took me to the edge of oblivion but, in another sense, they saved me. Without my bad habits delivering me to a state of desperation, and subsequently seeking help, I might never have discovered a better way of life. Recovery from addiction is about more than just giving up drink and drugs. That's just the start. The real work is in reflecting on your feelings, acknowledging your pain, understanding where it all comes from and learning to deal with it. Deal with it yourself, unaided by alcohol and drugs – or any other form of short-term, quick-fix distraction.

This book isn't just about addiction and recovery. You might not have any issues with drink or drugs. They just happened to play a big part in my mental health 'story'. Really, this book is about learning to deal with the shitty feelings and thoughts that bother all of us from time to time. Yes, even Jack the Lads like me. Maybe especially the likes of us.

We all face mental health challenges but not all of us can relate to all the airy-fairy 'wellness' chat. Wellness, I'm sure, has helped a ton of people but it's an industry. It makes money. And the discourse that surrounds that industry – the trite Instagram memes, the faux spirituality, the yoga-speak, the focus on vague concepts like 'manifesting' and 'abundance' – can be off-putting to many of us. I'm all for that stuff if it helps others. But I think we need lots of different ways of opening people up to conversations about mental health. We need to widen the vocabulary in order to widen the appeal.

The sort of blokes I've grown up with have generally used pride, resilience, humour and banter to form a cast-iron protective shield around their feelings. I think this is a problem. If we don't hear other men we can relate to being honest about their feelings and vulnerabilities, then we continue to think of ourselves as alone and isolated in our own world of pain. We assume everyone else has got things sussed apart from us. This can lead to feelings of shame and embarrassment that only make the bad feelings even worse.

Secrecy about our mental health issues can be extremely dangerous. Suicide is a big problem; it remains the biggest killer of men under the age of forty-five in the UK. Thank God I have never lost anyone close to me this way. But over the past ten years there have been a number of men within my broader sphere – ex-colleagues, friends of friends – who have taken their own lives. In each case, I learned it had happened suddenly and without any warning signs. These men hadn't spoken out about their struggles. In most cases, these men were loud and brash and fun loving; the last sort of blokes you would imagine were wrestling with self-doubt or misery. They were lads. Men like me and most of my mates. Maybe they thought those struggles didn't warrant discussion. But clearly, they did.

Speaking out needs to be normalised for every type of bloke. There needs to be as many different voices as possible out there describing these feelings and discussing ways of coping with them.

If you met me you'd probably think I was an over-confident loudmouth who never lost a wink of sleep to self-doubt in his life. Yes, I do come across as self-confident. I do spend a lot of time laughing, taking the piss, and presenting a carefree persona to the world. But I've had depression. I've lived with anxiety my whole life. I've had years of treatment for drink problems. I used to have a problem with cocaine and I've been taking anti-depressants every day for over a decade. And I used to be ashamed of all this. Now I couldn't give a fuck who knows about it. Quite the opposite: I am proud to have had the balls to face up to my problems and do something practical about them. I hope that by sharing this stuff, it might resonate with others and make them feel less alone.

I am not an expert and I don't want you to read this book as if it is a manual. It's not even advice, really. It's just an honest account of what I have gone through as an ordinary bloke with ordinary problems who has had to wrestle with ordinary pain. I want to tell you about it so perhaps, if you're going through anything similar, you will understand that you are not alone and it's nothing to be ashamed of. Maybe you will read about how I managed to get through the bad times and start to believe that you will do the same, however crap things might seem right now. I'm not going to tell you to 'stay positive' because I know how impossible that can be in the dark times. But I will tell you that you are tough enough to get through those dark times and come out stronger. You're stronger than you think.

Here's a couple of other things I need to mention right from the get-go. Firstly, and I can't stress this enough, I am a white, heterosexual, middle-aged bloke who lives a middle-class lifestyle in a nice part of a wealthy country. I have multiple advantages over 99 per cent of everyone else in the world. I do not think my problems or feelings are more special than anyone else's. So when I write about how much of a struggle it is to be a superlad who grew up hiding his feelings, don't for a minute think that I am saying people like me deserve any special treatment from anyone other than ourselves. This isn't a book about trying to change the world. It's a book about trying to change the way in which we as individuals can change our responses to the world. I am not interested in calling for men's rights. I don't think men like me need more rights, to be honest. Share some of them out to the marginalised, I say. And the same goes for when I write about fatherhood and how tough it can be. Is it tougher than motherhood? No. But so what? There are other books for mums. I'm a dad and that's the only experience I can write about with any authenticity.

These are my caveats. Straight white blokes like me are privileged in all sorts of very real ways, but feelings are feelings. Socioeconomic advantages don't incubate any of us from the experience of being human. All humans are vulnerable to feeling shit sometimes. I'm writing for men like me because that's all I'm qualified to do. Of course, this book might help mums, daughters, sisters, girlfriends and wives better understand what the men in their lives are going through too. If so, I'd be delighted about that.

I have divided this book into two parts: 'drunk' and 'sober'. Part one is about drunk me. I write about the stuff that shaped me in childhood and young adulthood; the things that I now regard as being fundamental to my sense of identity and the problems I faced as I got older. It's not all bad stuff – my childhood definitely had more positives than negatives – but I want to demonstrate that those early experiences can wind up dictating the way in which you respond to the world around you as you grow up. Even the little things can have a bigger influence than you might think. All of those early experiences in my life contributed to the crisis I underwent in my mid to late thirties, when I lost the thread. I started to get pretty bad bouts of depression and then started to drink and take drugs in a misguided attempt to stave it off. I now realise that a great deal of those problems were the result of me never really taking my mental health seriously and just ignoring all the little sources of pain and insecurity that had impacted upon me in the past.

Part two is about why I got sober, and how. That started for me in June 2015 when I went to seek professional help for the bad habits, which I had finally accepted were addictions. Only once I started to get on top of that stuff was I able to start addressing the deeper issues that had plagued me my entire life. Part two is about the way in which I live my life these days, with daily habits and attitudes that have made life so much more enjoyable than it used to be. It paints a picture of a life that is by no means perfect but is sunnier and more enjoyable now that I take my mental health more seriously.

I might lapse into offering advice throughout this book. Please try to ignore it. All I want to do is demonstrate my own vulnerabilities and tell you a bit about how I overcame them. To show you that you are not alone. And hopefully encourage you to take care of yourself a bit better.

PART 1
DRUNK

1

How to Pretend to Be OK

When I was two years old I burned myself severely. My mum had left one of my milk bottles sterilising by the sink. She was distracted for a split second and didn't see me reach up and grab it. The lid was loose, and the scalding-hot water splashed all over my arm. I screamed my head off as the skin peeled away from my flesh. My mum flew into a panic, an ambulance was called, and I was rushed to hospital where they had to give me a skin graft. They took skin off my arse and stuck it on to my mutated arm. The appearance was affected for ever. The entire inside of my right forearm was warped and mottled. The skin was bumpy and stretched. It looked like the lumpy skin that forms on the surface of cold porridge. When I started school a couple of years later, I dreaded T-shirt weather because the other kids would laugh at me for what they called my 'spaz arm'. These days, I still use the scarring – which now occupies a much smaller part of my arm – to help me differentiate between left and right.

Does this count as childhood trauma? Is it one of those repressed memories that I never think about consciously but in some imperceptible way shapes my worldview and dictates my emotional responses? Possibly, a little bit. Life is full of little incidents that hurt us. Part of getting to grips with your mental health is reflecting on all those little incidents and recognising them for what they were. I think most of us learn from an early age how to pretend to be OK and not make a fuss. We become brilliant at brushing things off. In a world where we are surrounded by constant reminders of extreme human tragedy – war, disease, famine, abuse, whatever – ordinary folk with ordinary problems can't allow themselves to view their ordinary pain as a legitimate source of trauma. But it really can be. Small moments of hurt, fear or shame can stay with you for ever if you choose to dismiss them as trivial. I'm not saying you need to make a big drama out of every little knock-back you ever get. But you at least should allow yourself to acknowledge your pain, however mundane it might seem. And to show yourself a bit of compassion when bad stuff happens to you. Mostly, young men are embarrassed to acknowledge their ordinary pain.

Someone once said to me, 'It's not the elephants that kill you, it's the ants.' It doesn't necessarily have to be something huge – like being the victim of abuse or seeing your best mate have his legs blown off by a landmine – that we label trauma. It might be something smaller, like mashing up your arm when you're a toddler. In fact, it can be even smaller stuff than that.

Not long after I burned my arm I was sitting on the steps in our front garden, minding my own business, looking at a line of ladybirds. My mum tells me I used to eat them. If that's true, I can't blame myself because ladybirds look like delicious sweets. So there I was, looking at – and perhaps nibbling on

– some ladybirds, when a tortoise wandered in through the front gate. I had never seen a tortoise before, even on TV. Imagine what a tortoise looks like to a child who has never previously seen one. It's like a tiny dinosaur. I screamed as badly as when I scalded my arm with boiling water. Apparently, it was a wild tortoise that roamed our estate. No one owned it. It relied on the kindness of strangers to give it food and shelter. The late seventies was a weird time. Was my encounter with it traumatising? Fuck yes. It's not just the ants and the elephants that will get you. It's the tortoises too.

In the mid-sixties my parents had three sons in the space of two and a half years. Theo, Dom and Cas were so close in age that they formed a particularly strong sibling bond. The family dynamic was well established when, seven years later, I suddenly turned up out of the blue. Whether I was a mistake or an attempted 'sticking plaster' baby designed to shore up a faltering marriage, I don't know. Either way, my parents split up shortly after my birth. There was a fairly significant generational gap between myself and my brothers. They must have been pretty surprised by my arrival but they never made me feel unwelcome.

I don't think my early years were a happy time for my family at all. My parents were splitting up and the home was filled with wild rows on a nightly basis. It wasn't a clean break up. There was a great deal of shouting, crying and emotional chaos. It's impossible that I wouldn't have been aware of it at the time, but it must have all been buried down in the depths of my mind. I was just a baby.

One day I came downstairs into the living room stark bollock naked. It's amazing how much time you spend wandering around naked when you're a kid, isn't it? My brothers, whom I completely idolised, all started screaming and pointing at me in horror. I freaked out and started to cry. 'Eurgh! What the fuck is that?' they shouted. They seemed to be fixated on my groin. My mum came in from the kitchen to see what all the fuss was about. 'Oh my God!' she screamed. 'It looks like a fucking egg!'

I peered down and, just as she had observed, a lump the size and shape of an egg was protruding from my groin. Burning flesh, miniature dinosaurs, aliens bursting out of my body: my whole early childhood was like a mad sci-fi horror. I know I am making it all sound a bit traumatising but, honestly, there was a great deal of love in my home too. I think I always understood that people cared about me. But the prevailing atmosphere was often a bit volatile.

The lump turned out to be a hernia, which eventually required surgery. In the meantime, it would appear from time to time without any warning, erupting from my groin and causing immense pain. Sometimes it would happen when I was at school. In the middle of playtime I would suddenly collapse, clutching my groin and crying my eyes out. What with that and my much-mocked 'spaz arm', I was quite the source of playground entertainment for a while. Whenever the hernia appeared my mum would be summoned to the school, and she would rush me to hospital where a doctor with a knack for these things would massage it into submission. I would be crying and screaming throughout – I can remember the pain vividly.

We lived in a small maisonette on a large council estate in Brentford, west London. After my dad left, my mum would have found it difficult to deal with the pain of the break up while also trying to corral three sons who were approaching adolescence and a fourth who was just out of nappies. The estate was a rough-and-tumble sort of place where kids (and tortoises) roamed free at night, dicking about and getting into trouble. I was still quite young when I started stumbling about the concrete alleyways, following my brothers around and observing what the bigger kids were getting up to.

One time I was walking back from the shops with my mum. A kid called Tyrone wandered up to us and shoved a peanut up my nose. My mum went crazy, and he ran off laughing. That peanut stayed up my nose for about a week until I eventually sneezed it out.

Life got pretty chaotic after my dad left. My mum was busy trying to juggle work while keeping an eye on the four of us in difficult circumstances. It was easy to go semi-feral. My brothers were at a tough age: trying to cope with the fallout from a divorce as they hurtled towards puberty, amidst the dubious temptations of a large council estate. Estates can be like little bubbles that trap their occupants, especially the younger ones, in a sort of parallel universe. Everything is incubated: the dramas, the hierarchies, the power dynamics. I was too young to remember most of it but it amplified the sense of instability and anxiety that had engulfed our family. Like most estates built in the post-war decades, it was cut off from the rest of the local community with its own pub and little parade of shops. My eldest brother Theo got a job in the Bejam where he would steal the fags he had started smoking prodigiously aged ten – not so much out of youthful rebellion as, I suspect, genuine need for some sort of stress outlet. He had been particularly close to my dad, who had moved to a smarter new apartment with a new girlfriend.

Theo started bunking off school regularly. Eventually he just stopped going altogether and ran away to stay with my grandparents in Hertfordshire. They lived in a small village called Chorleywood which, despite being only an hour outside London at the end of the Metropolitan line, felt to us like deepest rural England. There was a giant common and loads of green space, a tiny cluster of quaint shops and rows of cosy bungalows that looked like they belonged to another era. My dad's parents lived in one of them. It was a gorgeous little home that seemed to take us back a few decades whenever we entered. It was neat and tidy, there was a large sloping garden with well-tended flowerbeds and a small kitchen that constantly exuded the aromas of my grandma's cooking. It couldn't have been more different from the estate, with its hazardous atmosphere, mess and confusion. It felt peaceful, safe and predictable. No wonder Theo chose to disappear there for a while. Life back home had just become one barmy event after another.

My youngest brother, Cas, with his blond hair, brown eyes and big smile, seemed to have somehow been born with the swaggering self-confidence of Rod Stewart. Like Theo, he didn't really care for school much – especially after my dad left. His response to the whole situation was maybe a little less reflective and a little more 'fuck you' than Theo's. He would bunk off school with his mates and get up to no good. One day, when he was just ten and should have been at primary school playing hopscotch, he got into the home of one of his mates when the parents were out and guzzled half the drinks cabinet. My mum got a call at work saying he had passed out. An ambulance was called, and he was taken to hospital. Somehow, social services were not alerted, and I doubt my mum told my dad about the incident.

I don't want any of this to suggest my mum was anything less than a loving and devoted parent. She couldn't have made us feel more loved. But the practical reality of being the single parent of four sons, three of whom had been spun into a state of emotional mayhem while the fourth (me) was barely old enough to wipe his own arse, must have been overwhelming. She couldn't afford not to work – she had to rely on friends and family to support her with childcare and put some faith in her sons to behave responsibly. Which, of course, they didn't.

As the eldest, Theo was often given responsibility for me when my mum was out at work. He'd use the opportunity of a parent-free home to invite round his mates for raucous afternoons of drinking and anarchy. This was the tail-end of punk and most of them wore spiked hair in lurid colours, torn T-shirts and sometimes even eyeliner. As a means of easy entertainment, they taught me to do profane impersonations of their favourite punk icons. When they shouted, 'Johnny Rotten!' I would sneer and make the 'wanker' sign with my hand. They would fall about laughing. Then they would shout 'Sid Vicious!' whereupon I would curl my lip and grab my crotch. Years later, when I was an adolescent and they were already parents in their late twenties, they would see me at weddings or parties and shout 'Johnny Rotten! Sid Vicious!' and I would instinctively trot out the old routines. And we would all laugh.

The truth is that I probably felt pretty anxious and insecure in that little house of ours in the middle of the day, no grown-ups around, fag smoke filling the air and a bunch of pissed-up, raucous teens going mental all around me. The fact that my Sex Pistol impersonations seemed to make them approve of me in some way must have been comforting. Thus began a lifetime of trying to win approval and a weird sense of safety through showing off and acting the twat. Oh well, at least I've managed to monetise it along the way. Not all childhood traumas are entirely destructive.

One day, our entire front garden caught fire. Someone set light to the large vine that sprawled across our fence. Firemen were called to stop the flames infiltrating the house and spreading to other properties. I remember being at the swimming baths with my mum, watching one of my brothers compete in the school swimming gala, when someone rushed in to tell us what was happening. When we got back home, we watched the flames encroach upon our home while dozens of neighbours gathered round like ghouls. My mum started to cry and then I did too. I was five and thought I was seeing the building I slept in, the one steadfast and reliable bit of our family life, burn down. Eventually they put the fire out and the police turned up to investigate. They concluded, quite casually according to my mum's recollections, that it was an act of arson. Someone on the estate was trying to burn the Delaneys' home. But who? The police didn't know and said they had no way of finding out. It was at this stage that my mum started to look for an escape and our GP asked the council to have us transferred off the estate.

But it wasn't all peanuts up the nose and arson attacks. Some of the people on that estate were nice. My best mate was Mat Brown, who lived a few houses up with his older sister Jane and parents Duncan and Margaret. Jane was my first crush. She once cajoled me into bed with her. It was all very innocent – we were both fully clothed, but I have powerful memories of how exciting and illicit it felt when she pulled the neckline of her T-shirt slightly aside and instructed me sternly: 'Kiss me on the shoulder.' I did, and it felt magic.

'What do you prefer, Sam, legs or bums?' It's funny the questions you remember being asked in your life. That one has stuck in my mind for the forty or so years since it was fired at me, in Mat Brown's front room, by his mum, Margaret. I've no idea what the context of her saucy question was, but I recall it being asked amidst the warm, daft, slightly riotous atmosphere that always seemed to permeate the Brown household. They were a nuclear family who ate and laughed together, went on Sunday drives in Duncan's Triumph Stag, kept the house tidy, had proper jobs, nice toys and all the other things I could see normal families had. It wasn't like they were much richer than us. They were just a more conventional unit. I liked spending time there but I did not like being asked for my preferences about the female body. But I do remember my response. I didn't splutter like you might expect; neither did I grumpily refuse to answer or attempt to laugh it off. I looked Margaret dead in the eye and fired back, with the utmost seriousness, 'Legs. I like ladies with long legs.' The whole family fell about and I felt the same sort of relief as when performing the Sex Pistols stuff for the lads.

Margaret was kind to my brothers too. When my brother Cas bunked off school she would let him in the house during the day to play on Mat's Scalextric and drink cups of tea. My mum was furious when she found out Margaret had been harbouring her truant son. But that was Cas: he could somehow charm his way into housewives' front rooms before he'd even started shaving.

As for Duncan Brown, he was something of a local legend who had a greater influence on my life than he ever knew. He was a stocky man with a gravelly cockney voice, incessant chuckle and the swagger of an East End villain. He was tough, funny, outgoing and rebellious. When we moved a few years later to a house next to the A4 dual carriageway, he would drive over to pick up Mat from play dates and just speed off the road, across the grass bank and park up directly outside our front door with a beep of the horn. He couldn't be arsed taking an assigned exit and driving round the houses in the conventional (or to rephrase it, 'legal') way. He was Duncan Brown, an East

End cowboy tearing it up in suburban west London. I thought he was an absolute fucking superstar.

Being an East Ender, he supported West Ham and passed his love for his local club on to Mat. In west London in the late seventies supporting West Ham, a club from the opposite side of the city, was almost as strange and certainly rarer than supporting a club from Manchester or Liverpool. But I was bedazzled by Duncan, Mat and the whole Brown family, who took me under their wing and offered a picture of family life that could be simultaneously stable and fun.

I was hooked from my first visit to Upton Park. I liked the fact that it felt a bit different to support an unglamorous, relatively unsuccessful club from a different part of town. We lived right next door to Griffin Park and Brentford would have been the only honest choice as a local club. But with their claret and blue kit, nutty supporters and heroic-looking stars like Trevor Brooking and Billy Bonds, West Ham seemed perversely exotic to me. Supporting them gave me a sense of identity that wasn't inextricably linked to my older brothers. Although one of them, Dom, started supporting West Ham too, West Ham felt very much like my thing. It won me the approval of Duncan Brown, which was something extremely high on my agenda, and helped form an extra special bond with Mat. When we started school we lured a couple of new mates, Ollie and William, into our little West Ham cult. Ollie still sits next to me and my son at West Ham home games to this day.

When we walked into the playground of our local primary school in our claret and blue scarves and sweat bands, a gang of Spurs supporters – obviously enamoured by the blanket coverage of hooliganism served up by the media at the time – offered to fight us. And maybe because we saw ourselves (mistakenly, in my case at least) as tougher than them because

24

we were from the estate, we took them on by ourselves. After swinging our little fists with great bravery and gusto, if not technique, we were split up by teachers and made to stand outside the headmaster's room in shame. The school caretaker, Mr Leeds, walked past and asked us what we'd done to land ourselves in trouble.

'We were fighting over football,' we told him.

'That's a daft thing to do,' said Mr Leeds. 'I love my football team but you don't see me going round offering to fight people about it.'

'Who do you support, sir?' we asked.

'Leeds,' he said.

We couldn't get our heads around the fact that Mr Leeds supported Leeds and clearly didn't see anything strange or coincidental about that. We all burst out in laughter – me, Mat and the Spurs fans we'd only just finished scrapping with. It was the funniest thing we'd ever heard – we were in pieces – snot, tears, the lot. I think it healed the emotional wounds of the fight that had just taken place and there was never any football violence in the playground again.

2

Tell Me about Your
Mum and Dad

Everyone in my house was in a state of trauma but perhaps couldn't acknowledge that to themselves or each other. Divorce was more and more common in that era as people of my parents' generation – who had got together in the sixties and embraced a very modern idea of freedom and individuality – decided that they didn't want to commit to the conservative lifestyle choices of their parents. In other words, there were a few ex-hippies telling themselves: *Fuck this, man, I don't wanna settle down with the girl I met when I was eighteen and a bunch of screaming kids! I want to have some fun! I deserve more!* If that's what my dad thought when he decided to up sticks and leave, I'm not judging him for it. I can see why he might have arrived at that sort of decision.

One of the things I am trying to say in this book is that fatherhood is hard; much harder than anyone will tell you. I was surprised by how demanding it was; those early years of exhaustion and stress saw my drinking spin out of control. So I can't really judge my dad too harshly for what he did at a similar age. I turned to drink; he turned to another woman. We were both probably suffering from the same sort of malaise – and both looking to outside forces to soothe us. We perhaps should have been looking more closely at our feelings and trying to unravel them rather than just distracting ourselves. But nothing was pointing either of us in the right direction. How did we know what to do?

It's especially hard being a dad if you commit to do it properly. And my dad always did that when we were young, even after he left. When my brothers were little, he was always in and out of unpredictable, poorly paid, slightly artsy employment – film extra, roadie, gallery assistant, freelance copywriter – and spent a great deal of time at home, feeding the kids, doing the school run, changing nappies while my mum was out doing secretarial work. They were permanently skint and switched homes and locations constantly, very often doing midnight flits from landlords they couldn't afford to pay – with the kids, the cats and the furniture hastily bundled into the back of a mate's jalopy.

It was tough. It must have been exhausting for both my mum and dad. They were smart and wanted to raise their kids properly, with intelligence and care, even if they didn't have the money to offer them a more traditionally stable, middle-class life. My parents had got together in their teens and had three kids by the time they were in their early twenties. As a result, maybe my dad felt he hadn't had a chance to experience even a little bit of carefree living. A short period of youthful weightlessness in which you only have to really feel responsible for yourself. Unencumbered by dependants, obligations and bills. I had that – he didn't. To be fair, neither did my mum. But when you hit a crisis, which I guess he must have done around his thirties, you just want an easy out. You stop being able to think about wrong and right or fair and unfair. You just feel so terrible that you want to embrace whatever will take the feeling away in the short term. It's like being a drug addict: when you're clucking for drugs, all you can think about is your next fix. You're not going to listen to tedious lectures about the pitfalls of narcotics or engage with the lengthy and difficult processes of rehabilitation. Your mind is completely taken over by pain and the frantic desire to alleviate it.

My dad has never opened up to me about what he really went through at that time in his life. The story is only told from the perspective of those he left behind. There is general acceptance among all of us – including him – that he was simply the villain of the piece. It's an easy enough narrative to cling to: man drags wife and kids through years of poverty and instability as he tries in vain to pursue a variety of ill-advised bohemian endeavours before suddenly selling out, starting a corporate business, making a few quid for the first time in his life and running off with a younger woman.

I've spent a great deal of my life buying into this superficial rendition of events. It was easier to see him as a pantomime baddie, my mum as the wronged heroine, me and my brothers as the hapless collateral damage and his second wife as some sort of heartless siren. But none of those things is quite true. Each of the characters in the story played deeper and more complex roles in what happened; each of them – including my dad and Linda, the woman he left us for (and who turned out to be a kind and enthusiastic sort of stepmum under tricky circumstances) – would have suffered an unimaginable amount of pain, regret, confusion and inner conflict.

My mum had it bad, that's for sure. She was up Shit Creek without a paddle and had to toil in low-paid, miserable jobs for the rest of her working life while she saw my dad suddenly stumble late into business success and live out the eighties and nineties in some sort of yuppie fantasy.

So it's a compelling story of good and bad if you want to look at it that way; but as I've got older and lived through my own challenges I have come to understand what might have driven him to make the decisions he did. As I know, guilt can sometimes prevent you from opening up about just how difficult things are.

Maybe he sees being cast as the bad guy as penance. Perhaps it makes him almost feel a bit better in some perverse way. But here's the thing: aside from all the mistakes he has made, I know that he loved all of us, including my mum. And that's why I'm sure that his life must have become a living hell when he decided to leave us. The torment must have been almost unbearable. The love and devotion he felt towards his family in constant conflict with the unwanted knowledge that he couldn't be happy if he stayed with us.

It's something that has never happened to me but now, at last, I can comprehend to a greater extent. Which makes it easier for me to process the fact that my dad left me when I was just a baby. I have no recollection of ever living with him.

My brothers have always indicated that I had an easier childhood than them because I was blissfully unaware of the break up and had never known anything other than our single-parent life. Which is partly true. I didn't experience the same trauma they did. But I never had a proper, full-time dad. I never had that bloke who sat and had dinner with me every night or took me to the football or gave me advice when bigger kids had bullied me at school. I had a weekend dad, yes. And as weekend dads go he was pretty good. He'd pick me up most Saturday mornings and we'd go to museums or the park and all that stuff. He took me on holiday lots of times and we shared great memories. But it's not the same as having someone as a permanent, reassuring presence in your life. I grasped around for role models my whole life – very often looking in the worse possible places.

After he started his own ad agency, my dad rode the wave of Thatcher's economic revolution and immersed himself ever deeper in the life of a fancy-pants media exec around town (he bought a flat in St John's Wood and, at one point, even drove a Bentley). We, meanwhile, continued to live a bog-standard working-class lifestyle. He gave my mum a bit of money but not enough to survive so she worked part-time at building firms as a secretary and, later, as a carer for the elderly. The only other working people in my house as I grew up were my mum's boyfriend Archie – a milkman – and my brother Dom, who left school at sixteen to become a postman. We ate beans on toast for tea and watched the soaps on our rented telly in a living room that was heated by a four-bar gas fire that had only two settings: cold as fuck or hotter than the sun. The dog would stand too close to it while we watched *Coronation Street* and the air would be filled with the stench of scorched fur.

My dad would sometimes take me out to fancy restaurants with his new friends at weekends and I would feel totally out of place. I wouldn't understand the menus, I felt ashamed of my crappy Mothercare clothes and increasingly chubby physique, and I would constantly strain to smooth out my council estate diction when I ordered my food. 'I wish you wouldn't speak in that accent,' my dad would say. 'Nobody will ever take you seriously if you go around dropping your Ts.' He'd grown up on an estate too but had seemingly worked hard to disguise

31

any traces of his background from his speaking voice, which sounds very posh. He seemed frustrated that I was unwilling or unable to work as hard as he had to alter my identity.

But that was my accent. Those were my clothes and that was my fat body, nurtured by a diet of Findus Crispy Pancakes, Wotsits and Mars bars that I munched in front of the telly with a nervous intensity that foreshadowed my later struggles with drugs and booze. I was who I was. And I didn't feel like I fitted in with his new life. He was kind to me and he never made me feel unloved. He was a good dad. But I did get the sense that he was slightly disappointed in the way I was turning out (maybe something that all kids feel sometimes). I often felt like saying: 'Not as disappointed as I am, mate!'

I didn't feel particularly comfortable in my own skin when I was a kid. I wished I was smarter, tougher, more sophisticated, more sporty, funny, athletic and confident. I didn't ever quite feel enough. There was something missing in my life. Stability was one of those things. But there was also something missing inside me. I felt like I wasn't really a proper, fully formed boy who impressed his dad and made him feel proud. This, by the way, is not an objective truth. I'm not saying this was how my dad really thought about me. It was just the way I felt. I felt like the fat, ugly, embarrassing kid from the failed first marriage. I have spoken about this feeling more publicly in recent years and found that there is a bunch of other men out there who grew up feeling the same way. We were the broken-home generation.

Through sharing my experiences with other blokes who went through the same thing, I discovered a few similarities in the way we all turned out. Several of us transitioned from awkward kids to larger-than-life adults. Perhaps compensating for the insecurities that held us back in our early years, something flipped when we hit early adulthood and we became almost aggressively self-confident and perhaps a little egotistical too. These traits, in turn, helped eventually to lead us down the path of substance abuse and addiction as we struggled to wrestle with ways to channel our desire to be loved and noticed.

This being a book about mental health, you might have been expecting a bunch of stuff about my relationship with my mum and dad. Before I ever went to therapy (more of which later), like many other people I assumed that a great deal of it would involve an inscrutable shrink trying to convince me that my mum and dad were a pair of wankers. That was one of the things that put me off: it seemed like a clichéd and easy explanation for my adult problems and, in any case, I love my parents. If feeling better about myself involved me having to feel worse about them, I wasn't interested.

What I learned when I was finally driven into the arms of therapy by alcoholism and desperation was that talking about this childhood stuff and my parents wasn't nearly as prevalent as I had assumed. Obviously, it does come up once in a while. But rather than make me think badly about my mum and dad, it has actually done the opposite: a better understanding of myself comes from a better understanding of human beings in general. Often we put our parents on pedestals and apply higher standards to them than anyone else. Which is unfair and unrealistic, but the natural result of the dependent relationship you have with them when you're a kid.

Learning more about myself has helped me see my own parents as humans just like me or anyone else, with all the same flaws, insecurities and unresolved childhood issues of their own. Like all of us, they were doing the best they could.

Healing my own emotional wounds has involved learning to show myself more compassion. I have learned to feel less shame about my flaws and failures, and forgive myself for my mistakes by understanding the reasons behind them. I've come to see how complex and emotional we all are and why that means we are bound to do stuff that seems irrational or self-defeating at times. I have also come to apply that same thinking to my parents. My dad left and, yes, I'm certain that affected me in several negative ways. But he didn't leave as an act of cruelty, and he didn't do it with flippancy either. Just as we went through pain, he did too. I try to focus on that: I love him for the kindness and love he has always shown me and try not to think too harshly about the times he made me feel like shit. There's no way he meant to, and life will always cause individuals, however pure their intentions, to grate against each other from time to time. It might be a bit of a bland existence if we never did, to be honest.

I was six when the council transferred us to the small, terraced house next to the dual carriageway, on the border of Chiswick and Hammersmith. My best mate was Del, who lived round the corner. Del's dad wasn't around either. When your dad isn't present it allows you to make up bullshit stories about them. Del and I exchanged a few of these. Both of claimed that our dads were multimillionaires. My dad made adverts for a living. His worked down the sewers.

Our favourite hobby was to go outside to the waste ground opposite our houses, perched on the side of the A4, and dig holes using dessert spoons. We told ourselves that we were digging a tunnel to Disneyland. When we were nine, Del disappeared for a week. When he returned he told me his dad had taken him to Disneyland on Concorde. He even said he'd flown over our street on the way there and spotted me out the window digging on my own. I remember thinking that sewage workers must have been on an improbably handsome wage. I also felt a bit betrayed because the tunnel had always been a shared project driven by our mutual ambition to visit Disneyland. Now he'd been there, I sensed he might be a bit less motivated to complete our grand engineering scheme. He was certainly full of superlative praise for his visit to the legendary theme park: he told me he'd gone on a big wheel that spun so fast that he spat while at the top and was hit in the face by his own saliva on the second time round. Wow.

Del and I were always encouraging each other to get up to no good. We soon graduated from digging holes and started doing edgier stuff like bombmaking. We would fill empty jam jars with vinegar and bicarbonate of soda and plant them in the path of people walking down our street. Sometimes we would time it perfectly so the eruption happened just as some uptight commuter walked past and they would jump out of their skin. Del and I would roll out of our hiding place in the bushes, pissing ourselves laughing. It was, of course, a horrible stunt that could have blinded someone. But I was starting to get a little kick out of doing stupid stuff like that. And, each day, I would discover new ways of being an unsociable little wanker.

Sometimes we would go out on our bikes doing 'drive-bys' on older, tougher kids. We would spot a gang of them hanging about on a street corner, like kids used to do back then, and we would shout from a safe distance: 'Oi, wankers!' When they turned to look at us we'd give them the Vs and shout, 'Get fucked!' then cycle off in a state of terrified hysteria. What a wonderful and invigorating waste of time.

Del and I ran away a few times on our bikes, cycling all the way down Chiswick High Road and eventually into another postcode with dreams of disappearing. But I would always end up losing my bottle and riding home. Despite the chaos we lived in, I liked home. He genuinely seemed more committed than me to escaping his home life, which I got the impression was a bit less stable than my own. His dad wasn't about, he had an older brother in the nick and his other big brother, Terry (self-given nickname: 'The Tel'), was another tearaway. He used to come round my house quite a lot to ask my mum out. Obviously, I thought this was pretty weird and assumed he had no chance until one day she got dolled up and went out on a date with him to a local pub. Mercifully, it never worked out between them (The Tel was about twenty years her junior) but I found the whole episode disconcerting. It was not the first or last time my mother's love-life would cause me to spin out with anxiety and a strange, creepy discomfort that I still can't quite put my finger on. She was lonely and sad – still traumatised by my dad's departure and various other deeply upsetting events in her younger life, which I was yet to find out about. But none of that would have occurred to me when I was a kid. My mum is a larger-than-life character with an incredible sense of humour. It's a corny thing to say, but she lights up a room. As a result, it was impossible to conceive of the fact she might be quite miserable and insecure a lot of the time. Children don't really have much of a grasp on nuance or context and aren't the best at spotting the subtle clues about someone's inner pain. My dad was absent, my brothers were fucking mad and so my mum was the only thing that represented any form of stability in my life. Whenever she went out on a date with a bloke or, as she went through phases of doing, going out to discos with her pals in a bid to meet men, I would be consumed by a sense of panic, rejection and dread.

She got really into mysticism for a while and I would always be dragged along when she and her mates visited clairvoyants, palm readers and the like. I vividly recall one Friday night up a tower block in Acton, inside the flat of someone claiming to be a qualified tarot reader. I was plonked in front of the TV watching *Dynasty* while my mum was having her fortune told. I peered over to see what was happening just as the 'lovers' card was produced. The image of a naked man and woman, bound together in congress by a coiled snake, was truly disturbing. 'Ooh,' squealed the tarot reader in excitement. 'You're gonna meet a man!' My mum seemed thrilled. I was disgusted.

To be honest, I was also slightly put out by the idea that my mum might have space in her life for anything other than taking care of me. How dare she! To be honest, I would make her life hell at times by throwing a shit fit when she was on her way out on a date. Sometimes, I would go so mental that she just couldn't bring herself to leave me with a babysitter (usually one of my brothers) and would cancel her rendezvous at the last minute. I knew what I was doing and, in retrospect, it was manipulative and cruel. But when you're a kid you just want love and any perceived threat to that will fill you with absolute terror. If my mum ran off with a new bloke, where would that leave me? I would spend a great deal of time creating worst-case scenarios in which an awful dickhead would move in with us and make me call him 'Dad'.

In the end, one of her boyfriends really did move in with us. This was the aforementioned Archie the milkman, but he never asked me to call him dad. He was from Edinburgh, and he had a bubble perm and a moustache like almost every Liverpool midfielder of the time. I found him very entertaining and personable. But he was an alcoholic who struggled to get on with my brothers. After about two years living with us, his position in the family became untenable after he stole some of Dom's raspberry-ripple ice cream out of the freezer. Dom, tired and hungry after a nightshift at the Post Office, lost his rag and threatened Archie with a carving knife. Archie punched him in the face, then left for a new life in Jersey. My mum paid his airfare just to get rid of him.

* * *

It was a crossroads in my life. My mum was working hard to raise me as a good lad. She drummed into me the importance of compassion and kindness. She railed against bullying and encouraged me to look out for the vulnerable kids at school. She had a huge heart, was always going out of her way for people and served as a great role model when it came to helping others. My brothers, all big hearted in their own peculiar ways, were having a rough adolescence. Divorce and disruption had hit them hard; I can't speak for them but I suppose that feelings of rejection, abandonment, insecurity and anger were what drove much of their behaviour during this period. I was still at primary school but they were teens who bunked off, smoked, drank, fought, took drugs and generally acted like pricks throughout the whole of the 1980s. I thought they were cool as fuck but they were often scary to be around.

Theo eventually went to live with my dad but the two younger ones – Dom and Cas – were left to serve as my part-time care-givers-cum-tormentors. They were rubbish babysitters who would fill their time with me by sniffing glue or fighting. These were brutal fights, where knives would sometimes get brandished and objects would be smashed over the head. Their mates would also sometimes start trouble. I became used to life being extremely volatile with bouts of violence or drug binges happening all of a sudden in the house, often when I was just sitting around minding my own business and trying to watch *Grange Hill*. Stanley knives were pulled by disturbed teenage visitors to my house on more than one occasion. It was frightening. My mum was at work most of the time and these confused, angry, hormonally unstable hooligans were often what passed for my only childcare. I don't blame my brothers for anything; they were going through their own shit. They had enough on their plates without having to serve as my de facto dads. Things were a mess, though. I don't doubt this era of my life was responsible for the relentless state of anxiety I found myself in for most of my adult life. My mind and body were constantly on amber alert.

My brothers became anti-role models. I could see how much their antics worried my mum and often found myself consoling her when they left her in a distraught state of tears. I decided I wanted to be a good lad for her sake. Meanwhile, my dad was attempting – as best he could, given the weekends-only nature of our relationship – to raise me as a young man of intelligence and creativity. He encouraged me to read books and take an interest in nature. He took me to museums and tried gently to steer me towards noble, enriching pastimes such as playing chess and reading poetry. I showed only half-hearted interest in that sort of thing. Convincing a kid like me to get involved in that stuff would have taken full-time commitment. In the week, all I did was watch telly and dick about with Del.

The problem was that I saw myself as having a black and white choice in life: I could either be a nerdy spod who nourished his mind and soul with art and beauty; or a rule-breaking tearaway with a heart of rock and a brain shaped like a football. I was, of course, wrong. I would like my own children to be able to draw wisdom and fulfilment from all of life's varied pleasures and cultural corners.

It takes balls to be more than one thing at once. Throughout your life, people will try to pigeonhole you as a predictable archetype. They don't want to accept that you can be both down to earth but sophisticated, boisterous but sensitive, clever but stupid, all at once. You will be encouraged by society to adopt a prefabricated identity and stick to it scrupulously or be labelled a phoney. Fuck that. Do what you want. I wasted years of my life not opening my heart and mind to all sorts of love, joy and beauty because I thought it would mean I'd have to hand in my Jack the Lad card. This is a conspiracy drummed up by society to stop normal blokes from venturing beyond the cultural traditions of the British class system. A great deal of mental health is tied to our sense of identity. Are we living up to who we really want to be? That's hard to do when your identity has been handed to you by society and not formed through your own free will. There are so many different types of bloke you are told to be. It's important to make your own mind up about that and screw what other people think or say.

And as for talking about your feelings? Perhaps the reason I can't stop doing that sort of thing nowadays is that I had so much stored up from childhood. I would never have admitted to being sad, let alone lonely or scared, back then.

When I was ten, my dad split up with his girlfriend for about a year. During that period of time, I allowed myself to believe that my parents might actually get back together. One night, my dad came round to show off his new car to us. Before he arrived my mum had asked us if we might give her some time alone with him. I took this as a sign that something had been reignited between them and my mind began to conjure a fantasy in which we all lived together in a smart and tidy home: my dad and mum would fall back in love, Theo would come back, Cas and Dom would start behaving themselves, and we would just be dead normal and happy. It seemed alluring and, for a moment in the mid-eighties, I foolishly convinced myself that it was possible.

And then one day my brother Cas came into my bedroom and announced casually that our dad was back together with Linda and that they were getting married. I was heartbroken. Not just because he had got back together with Linda and arranged to marry her in such a sudden and dramatic way (that was his business, not mine, and she was a perfectly nice person who was always very kind to me), but because my dad hadn't bothered to tell me himself. I felt as if it couldn't be true if he hadn't told me about it.

After taking a moment to absorb the news, I burst out crying and didn't stop for quite a long time. It remains one of the most memorable cries of my life. On and on it went, the snot and tears spewing out of my face, and despite my abject embarrassment, I was completely unable to stop. Cas regarded me quizzically. 'Why are you crying?' he asked. 'I don't know,' I sobbed. And I think that was true.

'I suppose you've heard the news about Linda and me by now?' my dad asked when we were in the car on our way to the museums a few weeks later. He was at the wheel, looking straight ahead.

'Erm . . . yes,' I mumbled, looking down at my lap.

There was a silence and we continued to edge through traffic.

Eventually he said: 'Also, she is pregnant so you will be having a little brother or sister . . . so that's good, isn't it?'

Life felt like it was moving pretty fast. The few certainties I had clung to over the first decade of my life were being stood on their head. I had a vision of a new little brother arriving in pantaloons and a velvet waistcoat, speaking Latin at the dining table while my father applauded his precocious sophistication. I would be sitting beside him in a nylon tracksuit, eating my fifteenth Penguin biscuit and asking if I could be excused to watch *The Price Is Right* with Leslie Crowther.

It didn't turn out that way. By the time my little sister, MJ, came along I'd managed to get my head around the matter. For some reason, the fact that she was a girl disarmed me. I fell in love with her quickly and, mercifully, she turned out not to be a wanker. In fact, she is the very best of all of us. Even though my dad split up with her mum when she was still pretty young, she has grown up to be not just wildly smart and successful but, irritatingly, kind and modest too. It would be infuriating if I wasn't so proud of her. Perhaps she is evidence that you really can get over all this childhood trauma stuff if you're intelligent enough. I just never was.

I can't remember how I received the invite to my dad and Linda's wedding but it certainly wasn't formal. I think one of my brothers mentioned it to my mum who began to panic about buying me an appropriate outfit. My dad bunged her some cash to get me a half-decent shirt. God knows how she felt taking me out shopping for clothes to wear to her ex-husband's wedding.

The ceremony took place at Chelsea Town Hall. I arrived with my brothers, who all seemed excited to get stuck into the free booze. I was eleven, so I was too young to drink my way through the day but too old to have a designated adult 'handler'. My dad was distracted by being the groom and my brothers were busy getting shitfaced. So I spent the day sitting alone in a corner nursing a Coke and watching my dad's glamorous new pals from the advertising industry have a high old time of it, getting smashed and air kissing each other. I was at my very fattest at the time. I had tried to eat my way through the previous few months of misery. I've seen photos of the day wherein I am a sheepish and tubby presence, usually in the corner of the frame, with a weird spiky hairdo and a candy-striped shirt that was a touch too small for my rotund frame. I look fucking miserable. I was fucking miserable.

As we left the registry office and people chucked rice and confetti over the happy couple's heads, my grandma spotted me shuffling along behind the main throng with tears welling in my eyes. I felt a lump swell in my throat and began to panic. No blushing bride needs a fat, unwanted stepkid bursting out in tears as they line up for the money shot on the steps of the town hall. It wasn't that I was upset about the marriage itself. I liked Linda. I was perhaps even happy for my dad. I was even ready to accept that my mum and dad were never going to reunite. But the glamour, the glitz, the trendy wankers I'd never met who seemed to be bezzies with my dad and his missus all of a sudden – it just all made me feel completely disconnected and lonely. My dad's best man was a bloke I had never met before. He delivered a speech describing a version of my dad I didn't recognise. Everyone in the crowd laughed like braying horses. No fucker talked to me all day. I felt insecure, out of place, lost and awkward. My nan grabbed me by the hand and smiled at me kindly. For a moment, I felt seen – and the tears started to recede from my eyes.

The panic was over for a short while. But the feelings of dislocation would hang around for a few more decades yet.

3

A Beginner's Guide to Boozing

I can't remember the first time I tried booze. Some addicts have vivid recollections of the way it made them feel; the immediate sense of release; the instant realisation that it offered them an escape from all of their discomforts. None of my memories are so profound. Drinking always seemed really cool and grown up to me. I didn't feel aware of any discomfort or pain that needed alleviating. I looked up to my brothers and I desperately wanted to be like them. And their lives seemed to revolve around booze.

Boozing never seemed like a way out of anything bad; it seemed like a way into something brilliant. I liked the idea of pints in the pub on Saturday night and cans in front of *The Big Match* on Sunday afternoon. Beer was a really important lifestyle accessory; an essential part of the identity I wanted to cultivate from a very early age. I liked football and I was impressed by the sort of blokes I saw at matches; I was entertained by the rough lads that my brothers would bring round the house; I was wide eyed and thrilled at all the noisy banter and bullshit; I liked the music my brothers played in their bedroom by Madness, the Specials, the Jam and the Clash. It all represented something tough, cool, fun and rebellious. And alcohol was clearly central to all of it.

Access to some of the things kids aren't supposed to have was very easy from an early age. I'll give you an example. My mum always laid on a really nice Christmas. We all woke up to bulging stockings at the end of our beds. Chocolate money, walnuts, satsumas, the usual stuff. My brothers always got ten fags and a Clipper lighter. On Christmas 1989, when I had reached fourteen, she put fags in mine too – even though I never smoked. I told her this but she thought I was just trying to act like a goody two shoes. 'It's Christmas, I don't mind if you have a fag.' I just shared them out among my brothers.

My mum was never a big boozer but my brothers and I saw the true meaning of Christmas as being all about legitimised daytime drinking.

We all set about getting fully wankered from morning onwards: on lager, Baileys, whisky, Stone's ginger wine – anything from the arsenal of booze, lovingly accumulated inside the 'Christmas cupboard' over the preceding weeks. Then we got stoned. By the time the Christmas pudding was finished my brothers would have been on the gak, but I was still a bit too young for that. By six o'clock, other people started to join the party. My best mate Ollie came round, dropped off by his dad, a well-known television game show host of the era.

My brother Dom had a new girlfriend called Polly who turned up with a gift for the rest of us. She was obviously trying to impress because the gift was a brand-new Italia '90 themed Subbuteo set.

Now, Subbuteo was banned in our household because of all the violence. We used to run a league among ourselves and a few mates every Sunday afternoon on the kitchen table. We took it very seriously – whenever the FA Cup final was played we made our mum dress up as the Queen and go along the line of little plastic players, pretending to shake their hand and make small talk with them. But the matches would almost always end in punches being thrown so my mum had packed it all up into the attic and forbidden us from ever playing again.

By 1989 the ban had been in place for a couple of years and we pleaded with Mum that we had all matured a great deal in the interim. Plus, it was Christmas, and I don't suppose she wanted to offend Polly by denying us the chance to play with her very thoughtful present. So, she said we could have just a couple of games.

Bear in mind, we had all been on the cans since 9 a.m. and three of the family had been topping up with cocaine since lunchtime.

It was never going to be a straightforward Subbuteo tournament.

So we set up the new gear, all chose a team and decided, 'Fuck it, let's create the whole of the Italia '90 World Cup from group stages onwards! We could stay up all night if we want! It's Christmas!'

Things progressed as you might expect any Christmas Day Subbuteo tournament between four paralytic brothers to progress. Conflict. Anger. Accusations. Cheating. Spillages. And the creeping spectre of violence hanging over proceedings constantly until, BANG! It all exploded during a tense quarter-final encounter between Italy and West Germany.

An offside decision was disputed, voices were raised, things were said that could not be unsaid, a can of Foster's was spilled on the imitation AstroTurf pitch and the first fist went flying. Within seconds a bona fide melee was in full swing. Polly started crying. Ollie started to laugh with a nervous hysteria. Bella, our dog, ate three of the West German midfielders who had fallen to the floor amidst the mayhem.

My mum tried to defuse the situation in the only way she knew how: by pretending to faint. When nobody paid any attention, she got back up and pretended to faint again.

Eventually, the chaos was punctured by the reappearance of Ollie's famous dad at the front door. 'Everything all right?' he asked, peering down the hallway towards the signs of pandemonium in the kitchen. 'All fine!' said my mum in her best *I'm just a normal mum with a normal family having a magical Christmas Day with absolutely no fighting or drugs-*type voice.

And so, the tournament was abandoned. Everyone started to drift away to pubs or other people's houses and eventually it was just me and my mum left. Her finishing off the Stone's ginger wine and falling asleep on the sofa; me minesweeping the dregs of lukewarm beer cans and smoking the dog ends of abandoned spliffs in front of *Jean de Florette* on BBC Two.

Christmas round ours was always noisy, never boring, and usually actually quite fun.

There was plenty of love, yes, but it was very rarely relaxing or peaceful. It's fair to say that between the ages of nought and nineteen I felt decidedly 'on-edge' every 25 December.

It was at Christmas time when I first started to have an inkling that I might be a bit mad. Back in the eighties, 'mad' was a powerful term reserved for only the most overtly strange people in society. We all knew a couple of mad people and regarded them with a mixture of pity and amusement.

My family had a number of certified fruit-loops in its orbit. My mum has a bigger heart than most, so our household was what might be referred to in today's vernacular as 'a safe space for the mentally ill and emotionally vulnerable'. Back then we called our house 'a magnet for nutters'.

The year after Subbuteo-gate, we invited an all-star cast of our very maddest associates over for Christmas lunch. First, there was Auntie Ella, an elderly relative whose eccentric, train-of-thought babble throughout our festive lunch alternated between wailing tearfully over her dead husband, Uncle Fred, then suddenly producing tins of mints from her handbag and offering them round the table with a beaming smile.

My brother's mate Jason was a giant, wild-looking and hugely charismatic drug addict who sat next to Auntie Ella at lunch, showing an uncanny affection and warmth towards this old lady he had never met before.

Then there was Alberto, our neighbour from the flats up the road. He was a Peruvian chef, a diagnosed schizophrenic whose innate mental health problem had been compounded a few years earlier when a kitchen colleague at the fancy hotel he worked in had spiked his tea with LSD. He started tripping and had just never seemed to come down.

We invited these people because they didn't have anywhere else to go. And we loved each of them, in different ways. But there was no denying that their behaviour was entertaining. I must stress, we didn't invite them for their entertainment value. But, if I am honest, it was a bonus.

All sounds a bit cruel, I know, but what we didn't under-stand at the time was that these people – the 'nutters', the 'basket cases', those who were 'out where the buses don't run' – were more like the rest of us than we realised. Or at least cared to acknowledge. Their conditions had names that could be found in medical dictionaries: senility, schizophrenia, addiction. So we could categorise them neatly as 'barmy' and regard them as completely distinct from the rest of us, who merrily drank, smoked, shouted, snorted, argued and fought our way through the festive season in the manner only truly sane and stable people can.

That year, on Christmas Eve, I hadn't slept all night.

That song 'Spanish Flea' by Herb Alpert and the Tijuana Brass just kept looping through my mind. Where had it come from? What did it mean? I don't know. But I'm telling you now, this was no whimsical, amusing earworm like when you say you can't stop whistling Jona Lewie's 'Stop the Cavalry'.

It was a serious mental episode. That song came from nowhere, launched itself into my brain as my head hit the pillow on 24 December 1990 and set up camp for nine long, agonising hours. It got louder and louder and ever more intense. I covered my ears. I tossed and turned. I fought back tears. It was very distressing. Then morning came and I didn't mention it to anyone. Because it sounded mad – and mad was one of the most embarrassing things you could be.

Once the high-octane excitement and hedonism of the twenty-fifth had passed I began to sink quite quickly into a dark place. It started out as standard anticlimactic sadness, then morphed, by New Year, into my first taste of existential malaise. Christmas was over, the fun was dead, the future was cold, uncertain and pointless. Those were the thoughts that haunted my adolescent mind, like dismal accompanying lyrics to a backing track of 'Spanish Flea'.

On the night of 1 January 1991 I couldn't sleep because the dark thoughts had started to completely overwhelm me.

I became short of breath and started to sweat profusely. I must have been in big trouble because I decided to try and distract myself by actually picking up the book I'd been given by my English teacher to read over Christmas: *Northanger*

Abbey by Jane Austen. But the more I read it, the more anxious I became. I might not have been in the best frame of mind to judge the book objectively, and I am aware that many regard it as a right rollicking read, but I bloody hate that novel.

In the end, I just got this thought locked in my head that I was going to grow up alone and that everyone I currently knew and cared about would die. It was weird. I couldn't sleep in my bed so I took my blanket and pillows out into the hallway and set up a makeshift bed on the landing. It was closer to my mum's room, which I figured would come in handy if I started dying and needed her assistance in the night.

Of course, I know now that what I was experiencing was my first panic attack.

The signs should have been clear that Christmas and New Year: I, too, was out where the buses didn't run. Not quite as far out as Auntie Ella or Jason or Alberto, maybe. My mental illness didn't have a proper name, not back then anyway. Maybe it would have been better if it had. Then I wouldn't have hidden it from everyone so studiously like a dirty secret. The mad thoughts I had, the scary voices in my head, the scattergun paranoia and the relentlessly irritating songs that plagued my nights just seemed stupid, embarrassing and trivial.

So, I did what I think 99 per cent of all people did back then: I learned how to pretend to be OK. And I got pretty good at that. I hid all the weird crap in my brain that was upsetting me. I figured it would eventually just go away. It didn't, it just got worse, and I had to get better at hiding it. If I'd been able to recognise it as an actual problem and talk to someone about it with honesty and an absence of shame, I might have been able to skip the bits of my life that came years later with the drugs, drink and therapy. It would have saved me a great deal of pain – not to mention a shedload of time and money.

A few months after that Christmas, Auntie Ella started shitting in her handbag. Then she died. Jason died that year, too, of a heroin overdose. I'm glad we at least got to give them both a bit of fun and laughter on what turned out to be their final Christmas.

Alberto is still very much around and remains a good mate, but his struggles continue to this day. I've got more understanding of what he has had to live with now.

I've learned that worries, periods of sadness and strange thoughts never go away completely. But you've got a better chance of staving them off if you acknowledge they exist. I feel sorry for fifteen-year-old me, lying in the hallway, terrified of his own thoughts but even more terrified of everybody talking about them to anyone. I felt alone and scared. The moment I chose to observe and accept my own madness, I finally assumed some power over it.

4

Fear and Self-loathing in West London

I have been mates with Joe since September 1986. That was the month I started secondary school – he was the first new pal I made there. Even at that tender age, Joe had chiselled good looks and a charming personality that had the girls in our year craving his attention. He was funny and, crucially, not in any sense a wanker (which, as we all know, is rare among the attractive and popular folk at school). So when he picked me out to be his mate I felt honoured, as if I were being touched by stardom.

Another thing about Joe was that his mum was head of the Parent Teacher Association. In my world, this was like having a mum who was the queen. My mum, lovely and attentive as she was, had a strangely intense cynicism towards the PTA, seeing it as an organisation for uptight snobs and hectoring poshies. She would use PTA as a term of abuse: in traffic she would shout things like 'Look at her in her fucking Volvo – typical PTA wanker.'

This meant that I felt intimidated by anyone who had a mum in the PTA. Like they were from a higher social order who looked down upon the rest of us. So, while it was quite exciting, being mates with Joe also felt quite pressurised. In short, I wasn't entirely sure I was good enough to exist in the thrilling glow of his orbit.

One day after school he came over to mine for tea. Because my mum was always at work and my brothers and I were disgusting, lazy slobs, our little house was always messy. So I felt a little bit ashamed welcoming mates round there, especially glamorous new ones like Joe.

But, like I say, he wasn't a wanker and didn't give me the slightest hint that he was appalled by the cheap furniture, dirty dishes or dog piss on the kitchen lino that greeted us when we walked through the door. Still, I couldn't shake the idea that he was just really good at hiding how horrified he was at my living conditions.

Nevertheless, he stayed for tea, met my mum and everything was going swimmingly. Until my brother Dom got in from his shift at the Post Office and started arguing with my mum about money. He was late with the housekeeping again. The argument escalated extremely quickly – as arguments in our household tended to do. Voices were raised, accusations were thrown, profanities were exchanged. Judging by the look on Joe's face as this all unfolded before him, I felt certain that he had never heard a mum call her son 'a lying wanker' before.

Tea that night was baked potato with beans and cheese. I was halfway through mine when Dom snatched it from the table and lobbed it across the room in rage. It smashed against the wall, orangey Heinz sauce splattering everywhere.

Then he stormed out of the house, got on his motorbike and disappeared. My mum, obviously needing a bit of a cool-down, followed him out the door and had a stomp round the block.

Alone in the house, Joe and I responded to the deeply awkward situation in the way that all young lads tend to: by completely ignoring it. I shut the front door and suggested we watched a bit of telly. He politely acted like nothing had happened. It was better that way. But then there was a knock at the door. It was Joe's mum – Joe's head-of-the-PTA mum! – come to pick him up.

FUCK! It was the stuff of farce. Like the vicar turning up for tea just as the dog has run off with your trousers. I tried to usher Joe out of the front door quickly so his mum wouldn't be exposed to the barmy innards of my home. But then she asked to meet my mum. 'Sorry, my mum's not here,' I muttered. She asked to meet my dad. 'My dad doesn't live here,' I said.

'Are there any adults here?'

'No . . . there were some. But, erm, they've all gone.'

I blushed. Joe looked at his feet. She was in the hallway now, peering into the kitchen where the broken plate lay in pieces all over the floor and the colourful components of my dinner clung to the walls.

She asked if I wanted her to wait with me until my mum got back. The gentle concern in her voice burned my cheeks with shame. I told her I was fine and that my mum would be back any minute. So they put me out of my misery and left. I started cleaning the kitchen.

I have this recurring dream where I'm doing a shit in public. It's plagued me for years. A while back, I told my therapist about it and she said it was probably associated with shame. I was confused at first because, amidst the plethora of mental irritations that bother me daily, shame was not one I was ever aware of. But then I dug a bit deeper and remembered the way I felt on the first time Joe came round my house. Beansgate,

I call it. It was not an unusual feeling for me back then. And I realised that the discomfort I sometimes felt about myself in adulthood – those feelings I tried to numb with booze, drugs or whatever other distraction I could find – might have been a continuation of that. A mild disgust at myself that I was always trying to hide from.

I often felt ashamed of myself, and of how and where I lived. I shouldn't have done because it was mostly a fun and happy place that was full of love. But I had plenty of mates who lived in bigger, smarter homes than mine with polite, well-spoken parents and siblings who seemed to get along and never threw their dinner at each other.

All of this added to the nagging sense I had that my dad always looked down on me. I don't think anyone was trying to make me feel ashamed. The feeling just existed in my head. An insecurity, a sense that I was less than other people, a desire to hide the parts of myself that were ugly or messy because I assumed that they would make people dislike me.

I was wrong about that when I was an awkward kid and I was still wrong about it when I was a drunken adult. Sobriety taught me that I was able to be my complete self – with the shit bits, the awkward bits, the ugly bits and the insecure bits all on display – and that people would still like me. Often they liked me even more because I carried myself with greater honesty. Not everyone, of course. Some people still think I'm a wanker. But that's OK. At least now they can make that judgement based on all the facts.

I went round to Joe's house a week after Beansgate. Turns out, it was just as messy as mine. They weren't posh at all. Joe might have been implausibly good looking and his mum a high flier in the PTA, but they were about as kind and down-to-earth as any family I've met before or since. They had loads of pets, including two talking parrots that shat everywhere. Plus Joe argued non-stop with his siblings, and his mum and stepdad shouted at them constantly. It was a right laugh. Their house was chaotic, noisy, fun and full of love. I felt right at home there.

The lesson in all of this was that everyone's life is messier than it seems. All the mates I had who lived in posher houses with seemingly more conventional families were all going through their own private problems behind the scenes. It took me years to understand that. I just always assumed that everyone else's life was perfect and that I had to hide the shitty bits of my own or they might not like me any more. But as someone smart once told me: 'Comparing is despairing.' Most people don't judge. Most people aren't even paying attention to your life – they're too tied up in their own crap. And those who do sneer aren't worth your time and energy anyway.

I was lucky to become friends with people like Joe – and the handful of other incredible people I met at school and who remain my closest pals to this day. But the strength of those friendships was not enough to combat the complex mental and emotional challenges that adolescence presented. In fact, my problems had only just begun: I was about to discover girls.

Every single time I went on a school trip I came back with a massive, all-consuming crush. I met a girl on a daytrip to France when I was twelve and fell in love before we got off the ferry in Dieppe. I couldn't believe she was showing me so much attention. I was naive enough to assume it meant we were more or less an item. But then we got back to school the following week and she ignored me.

A few weeks later she took me aside in the playground and told me she had started dating a notorious fifteen-year-old psychopath who looked easily big and grizzled enough to be on the pro-darts circuit.

I didn't really understand why she made such a special effort to break the news to me about her love affair with the school lunatic. I just remember clearing my throat and saying 'congratulations' in an involuntarily high-pitched squeak. Inside, my heart quietly broke for the first time.

A couple of days later I came face-to-face with the psycho in question.

He was walking into the art block as I was walking out, accidentally blocking his path. He looked me up and down, something seemed to register in his eyes, and he punched me so hard in the chest that I literally took off and flew back into the building, crashing against a wall.

I brushed it off. I'm not trying to boast or anything. Mine was the sort of school where being smashed into a wall by a child-man on your way from art to double physics was not that unusual.

I was actually quite flattered at the time. I took his act of completely disproportionate violence (I mean, he could have just said 'excuse me') to be evidence that I was regarded as a serious love rival. As I was sitting wheezing on the floor of the art block, waiting for the air to return to my lungs and for the other kids to stop laughing at me, I allowed myself a small sense of self-satisfaction.

We've all got a bunch of stories about teenage heartbreak and humiliation. I used to think I had more than most but then I started sharing them with pals to make them laugh and they would share back. It became like a perverse contest to see which of us had been the most useless and unlucky in love.

I've got loads of those memories. Once, a couple of years later, another girl I had a crush on split up with her boyfriend and, while presumably on the rebound, asked me if I'd join her on a week's holiday in Wales at one of those organised summer adventure camps.

A week's holiday with the girl of my dreams? When I was just fourteen? Yes, I thought my ship had well and truly come in. We travelled to the Brecon Beacons together on a coach and, on arrival at our secure compound for Outward Bound teens, we were spilt up into separate boys and girls dorms. Although we were not officially boyfriend and girlfriend yet, I confidently assumed that we would be meeting on neutral ground later that day for some fairly robust French kissing.

That night there was a welcome disco for all the kids.

I attended with my new dorm-mate, a lad from East Grinstead called Aaron whom I'd met hours previously. When we got there I introduced him to my de facto girlfriend and the pair of them hit it off right away. In fact, after a couple of dances, they disappeared with each other completely for about forty minutes. On their return, they announced they were now 'going out' with each other. Laugh? I almost called my mum from the payphone to ask if she'd come and collect me.

Instead, I spent a lonely and miserable week in the damp Welsh countryside, reluctantly taking part in orienteering exercises while watching Aaron French kiss the girl I had come there with. Don't cry for me. I was just a lad who loved too much.

Getting this stuff off my chest is cathartic. It helps to turn the micro-tragedies of your past into comic anecdotes wherever you can. It takes the sting out of them. Because all of them do sting. Yes, they are funny in retrospect but all those little dramas leave their scars. Most of us are too proud to admit that to ourselves – let alone anyone else – at the time. But delving back into the little moments that hurt you during those formative years can be helpful. It's not just the big traumas that shape your emotional responses to the world. It's the little papercuts you suffer along the way and never really confront.

It seems pretty stupid and arduous to audit all of those little moments of forgotten pain. But the point is to acknowledge that all of the little bruises you pick up through life can accumulate into bigger wounds. Did the seemingly inconsequential liaisons of my youth contribute, in some tiny way, to my eventually developing a batshit booze-and-charlie habit in my thirties? Or was it something to do with my dad leaving, or my mum dating the milkman, or my older brothers locking me in the airing cupboard? Or was it none of those things? Did I simply love getting on the beer and gak so much that I just couldn't stop before it was almost too late? Fuck knows, to be honest. Maybe a combination of all those things. Or maybe I was just born a twat.

What I do know is that acknowledging pain or sadness when it happens is important.

Rather than worrying about losing face, you should realise that the tougher thing to do is hold your hands up and say: 'That's right, lads, I've had an absolute nightmare and – to be honest – I could do with a cuddle.'

Hiding the way you feel is exhausting and makes everything so much harder. You'll never move on if you spend all your time worrying about appearing cool or unflappable. It's pretty transparent when people put on that sort of act anyway. I happen to think that overt displays of pride are for uptight dickheads who haven't got the balls to ask for help.

We've all had crap times, big and small. Lying about their significance to yourself or others is a waste of energy. These days, I prefer to own that shit.

5

How to Hate Yourself

When I was in the fifth year at secondary school, we'd play football every Friday afternoon. The PE teacher would let us wear our own kit and just leave us to it for an hour. It was a great way to end the week. One Friday when I was sixteen – just a few weeks from leaving the school for good – I was warming up before kick-off by taking a few shots at the goalie. We had been separated as usual into team bibs and team no-bibs. I was lucky enough to be on the bibs side with the school's best footballer, Alan Henderson. Alan was also the hardest kid in the school. He was the sort of lad who'd looked and acted like a twenty-five-year-old middleweight boxer since he was eleven. He was quiet and moody and we all regarded him as a celebrity. The fact that I was warming up with him prior to kick-off felt, in itself, like an honour. I passed the ball to Alan and he thundered it into the back of the net. He then took the ball back from the keeper and teed me up for a shot. In a state of nervous excitement, desperate to impress him, I panicked, leaned back and completely spooned it. It not only cleared the goal but actually went over the ten-foot-high fence that surrounded the pitch. It was a shot so badly executed that it almost orbited the fucking moon. Eventually, the ball bounced and settled by a kerb in the road outside the school.

'Fucking idiot,' snarled Alan Henderson, justifiably. 'Go and get it.' So off I jogged in the direction of the school gates. But Alan was impatient. 'No, don't run all the way round,' he said. 'Just climb over the fence and get it.'

I didn't really fancy the climb. The fence was tall and intimidating and everyone was watching. But when Alan Henderson ordered you to do something, you had to do it. So up I went, scaling the wire mesh fairly easily until I got to the top and swung my leg over to the other side. Suddenly, I couldn't move. My shorts (which were quite baggy, as was the style of the time) had caught on a protruding piece of wire. I clung to the fence with both hands to keep myself steady. I let go with one hand to try and untangle myself but immediately lost balance. So I just sat there, clinging anxiously to the top of the fence. I don't know if you've ever been stuck up a ten-foot-high fence but I can tell you, when you're looking down, it feels more like fifty feet.

'What the fuck are you doing?' barked Alan Henderson.

'I'm stuck!' I whimpered.

Suddenly, Henderson was joined by Mr Kitson, the unscrupulous PE teacher.

'What the fuck are you doing?' he echoed.

'My shorts are caught on the wire, sir. I can't unhook them!'

'Well what are you wearing such baggy shorts for? You look ridiculous!' he shouted.

'Yes, sir,' I replied.

By this stage, all of the other lads had gathered at the foot of the fence. Naturally, they all found my predicament hysterical.

Mr Kitson refused to climb up and rescue me because, he said, it was all my own fault. Instead, he sent someone to get a replacement ball from the sports hall and just left me to watch the game from my vantage point up on the big fence, like I was an umpire at Wimbledon. What made all of this worse was that all the girls in my year were playing netball on the adjoining pitch. Soon they noticed what was going on. 'What are you doing, Sam?' they asked.

'Just watching the game,' I said.

I was trying to be casual about it – like I had actually decided to watch from up on the fence. But they had my number. As I was sitting there, terrified of falling, being laughed at and teased by these girls – many of whom I had crushes on – and watching the other lads get on with the match, I felt as if my entire school career had been encapsulated in one neat predicament.

Eventually, once the match was over and everyone had gone back into the changing rooms, one of my mates finally took pity on me and climbed up to help unhook my shorts.

I'd like to tell you that was the most embarrassing PE lesson of my life. But I'm not certain it was. I was no stranger to indignity at that age. I was never particularly sporty, clever or tough. So things weren't always easy. Despite that, I look back on my school days with mostly happy memories. The people I met there were smart and funny. It's where I met Anna, the girl I would eventually marry. My best mates today are still the lads I hung around with at school. We didn't learn a great deal but we had a good laugh. And despite my athletic and academic shortcomings, I had one huge advantage: self-confidence. From day one, I felt able to stand up for myself when necessary and show off constantly. Maybe it was the result of being from such a large, noisy family. I was used to standing up to older brothers and holding my own with people much older than me. So other kids – even the psychopathic kind, of which we had a few at my school – were not particularly intimidating to me. I wouldn't have been able to fight them but I could usually talk my way out of tight spots. I certainly didn't feel quite so confident on the inside but, on the outside, I was brilliant at faking it. I revelled in standing up to petty-minded, belligerent teachers. As a result, I often found myself in more trouble than the naughty kids who were always fighting, smoking or bunking off. I always showed up at school and usually got my homework done on time. But I think most of the teachers thought I was a fucking pain in the arse.

I grew up besotted with the American high-school movies like *Pretty in Pink*, *Weird Science* and *Ferris Bueller's Day Off*. They made school seem so much more glamorous than it was in dreary old England. The kids were beautiful, they didn't have to wear uniforms and they all drove to school in their own cars. Perhaps just as appealing was the neat order of their social hierarchies. There were jocks and nerds; cool kids and losers; mathletes and cheerleaders. As British kids who devoured these films on VHS we had more understanding of the archetypes at American schools than we did our own.

I'm not sure anyone in my school fitted quite so well into any of those groups. All of us resided in a complex and ever-shifting social Venn diagram.

My brothers had all been bombed out of the local comprehensive so I was sent to one with a slightly better reputation a few postcodes away. It was a state school, but it was smaller and in a slightly leafier part of the suburbs. Nevertheless, it was a real social mix: some kids from nearby estates, others from the large, smart houses that surrounded the school. It was racially and socially diverse – which seemed perfectly normal to me at the time. It's only as I got older that I began to realise much of the world was divided up into various ghettos, both good and bad. I've always felt privileged to have been educated in such a diverse environment. I think it gave all of us who went there the confidence to traverse all sorts of different social circles with a self-assurance that you sometimes see lacking in the privately educated. The cliché is that public schools breed adults with cast-iron confidence. But when I grew up and joined the media industry, which is dominated by the privately educated, I noted how awkward and nervy these posh people became when they found themselves having to talk to someone from outside their own circles. It didn't seem to hold them back too much – but that's because the industries they worked in were full of people just like them. Have you ever seen someone from a posh school having to ride the bus, talk to black people or make themselves a sandwich? It can be fucking embarrassing.

When I look back I realise my school was a madhouse, just like all secondary schools. Schools are barmy: filled with people going through probably the most confusing and scary five years of their lives. Personalities and hormones are all over the place. Everyone is trying to find an identity, often changing it from one day to the next. Everyone is going through their own secret dramas at home, which they are desperately trying to hide. At a mixed school like mine, we all spent a huge amount of time and energy wrestling with debilitating crushes, sexual insecurities and suffocating social anxiety. But none of that was spoken about explicitly because we were so embarrassed by it. The teachers had to pretend to themselves and the students that the whole purpose was academic learning. But that was a side show: we were all trying to squeeze education in around the edges of our real preoccupations, which were entirely emotional.

So many of the kids were oddballs. There was one boy known only as RoboCop because he moved and spoke entirely like the hero of the popular action flick of the time. He committed to this characterisation fully. Even in lessons, he would answer the teacher's questions in a robotic, American voice and frequently pretend to be drawing a pistol from his imaginary leg armour. There was another lad who thought he was a car, moving between classrooms to the sound of his own engine noises, even changing gears with an imaginary gear stick.

There was a kid in my tutor groups called Gary who was obsessed with Elvis. He had the balls to come in on the first day with a huge quiff that stank of Brylcreem and a denim jacket with the collar turned up. This was 1986. 'What's with the quiff, mate?' we asked him. He curled his lip and replied in a perfect Memphis drawl: 'That there's my Elvis hair.' He accompanied this with a little hip thrust and knee twist. Astounding. Now there was a kid who had selected his own identity and was entirely at ease with it from day one. He continued this routine for the next five years. Every school day until we left in the summer of 1991 he turned up with the same hair and jacket, speaking almost entirely in Elvis. He got the piss taken out of him for about the first month until we realised he wasn't going to give up and then everyone just got used to it. His best-ever moment was when the teacher asked him what he was planning on having for lunch one day and he got up out of his chair, walked up to the front of the class and, in a beautifully ostentatious Elvis impersonation, bellowed: 'Baked potato, beans, cheese and buuuuuutteeeeerrrr!' while doing the full Las Vegas karate routine. We actually applauded that. What a glorious weirdo.

The school was full of them. The day after the famous storms that swept through London in 1987, I went down to the local park with a couple of mates in our lunchbreak to survey the damage. Two very large trees had fallen from opposite sides of a stream, leaning into each other and making an upside-down V-shape over the water. When you're a bored kid you conjure the most superbly idiotic ways to waste time and just throw them about as if they are part of normal conversation. 'I bet you a fiver you won't climb up to the top of them trees and shit into the stream,' I said to my mate Mark, who was pretty mental and always up for a laugh.

'All right, you're on,' he said without hesitation.

So up he climbed, about fifteen feet to the top of this tree formation. At the top he called out to the rest of us: 'Can you see me from the park?' We walked back as far as we could and shouted back: 'Nah, you're hidden by all the other trees. Go for it, mate!'

This was bollocks. He was completely exposed and everyone else in the park could see him. He started to undo his trousers and pull down his pants. We summoned all the other kids in the park over, explaining that someone was about to shit into the stream. Sure enough, Mark delivered on his promise. It was one of the most extraordinary spectacles I have ever witnessed. But not everyone was as impressed as I was. A group of rough fifth years were so disgusted by what they had seen that they resolved to dish out a punishment beating. 'Do you know that kid?' they asked me angrily. To my shame, I told them I did not. When Mark climbed back down the tree they chased him all the way back to the school gates. He hadn't even time to wipe his arse with a dock leaf.

These are all typical, fun stories but, looking back on it now, this type of behaviour seems to have been indicative of a mental health crisis inside the school. My school was nothing special. It wasn't any rougher or run down than the next state-funded institution during the Thatcher era. I'm pretty sure anyone reading this would, if they thought back hard enough, be able to recall incidents just as weird and characters just as peculiar as Little Elvis and Tree Shitter Mark. Schools are hives of mass, unaddressed mental illness. At least they were back then. They've all got mental health lessons and counsellors coming out of their ears these days, which is great.

By the third year (what they call year nine these days) at least half the year were boozing and smoking weed, at least at the weekends. I had been desperate to get stuck into pub culture from the age of ten, when my brothers used to sometimes bring me in the local for a Coke. I associated going down the pub with being a proper lad. When my brothers all piled back in the house after closing time, smelling of beer, laughing their heads off and babbling nonsense, I would look at them and think: *Wow, being grown up looks like the best fun in the world!*

Yep, my horizons were set pretty low.

But I had to wait for the pub. In the meantime, me and my mates made do with warm cans of beer stolen from our parents and guzzled down the park. The first time I remember getting properly wankered was New Year's Eve when I was thirteen. My brother Theo's birthday is on New Year's Eve and he'd thrown a party to celebrate. Me and my mate Joe nicked a bottle of tequila and drank an excessive amount up in my bedroom, wincing at the vile flavour as it stung our throats. We then snuck out for a badly rolled joint on the benches at the top of my road. When I got back to the house, drunk, stoned, nauseous and completely disorientated, I started to vomit everywhere. In the hallway, all the way up the stairs and into my bedroom, where I lay, spewing into old tea mugs and groaning, 'I am dying.' I remember Theo finding me there and laughing: 'It's fine, mate, you're not going to die. You just want to die.' He was right, I did.

Getting spannered like that became a weekend habit for me and everyone I knew. I began to become conscious of the kids who were cool and popular, and wanted to be part of that gang. They were into music and went to parties at weekends. I was into football which, in the 1980s, was decidedly not cool. This was the era of hooliganism, Hillsborough and Heysel. Before Italia '90, Euro '96, the Premier League, Sky TV and the rehabilitation of football's 'brand', it went through a phase of being regarded as a washed-up sport played by weird blokes with bad haircuts and watched by racists, homophobes and psychopaths. This wasn't an entirely accurate picture (although there were some kernels of truth in it) but it was certainly the way it was portrayed by much of the media and perceived by people who weren't in the know. But I never took a break from my all-consuming addiction to the game and spent most of my time either thinking about it, talking about it or playing it with my mates, predominantly my old pal from primary school, Ollie. We both loved West Ham. His dad Steve would take us when we were younger but when we were twelve we started getting the train over to Upton Park by ourselves.

Back then, being one of the football lads almost precluded you from being in the cool gang. I had a mate who started dating one of the coolest girls in the school, but he was rejected by her social circle because of the fact he played in the school football team. So he was forced to make a decision and, understandably, chose the girl. He quit the football team – but she dumped him for another bloke a few weeks later anyway. By which time the team coach had the hump and refused to reinstate him. Gutted.

When I did manage to get into parties at the weekend I would try to cement my credentials as one of the cool kids by drinking as heavily as possible. It became clear from an early age that making a drunken spectacle of yourself at the weekend was not so much a source of humiliation as valuable social currency. If you threw up at the park from smoking a bucket bong or downing a load of Southern Comfort (the teenage choice of the time) then people would talk about you at school on Monday like you were a rock star. Drunken indignity doesn't always get the negative feedback it deserves. When you're young, it's a badge of honour.

When I look back I can see how booze was working its way into the fabric of my life so insidiously. Adolescence is a very confusing time, filled with anxieties and insecurity, and booze presented itself so readily as a solution. Culturally, it was all around me: the cools kids at school drank it, my older role models drank it, the rough lads I looked up to at football drank it. You were bombarded with alluring impressions of booze and the cool, tough, fun-loving and attractive person it made you. I didn't drink to 'forget'. I drank to show off and have fun. But subconsciously booze was working its way into my heart and mind; I was learning to use it as a crutch in so many different aspects of my life. Eventually, I would come to depend on it to get through the day. But by that stage it was almost too late. In those early days of fun-filled rebellion, alcohol was like a wolf in sheep's clothing.

There were so many sources of anxiety at the time; so many reasons to feel uncomfortable or worried. In early adolescence I was still dead insecure about my looks. At home, my brothers gave me constant grief for being chubby. They would shout 'doughnuts' at me whenever I walked in the room. One time, my dad even took my mum aside to complain about my increasingly chubby form. He said it was unhealthy and that it was her responsibility to do something about it. I know this because, for some reason, she chose to report the whole conversation back to me straight after he'd left.

My mum was never cruel, just pathologically unable to keep her mouth shut. She had no filter, and was unable to hide her feelings and anxieties from her children even when it would have been much better for everyone if she had done so.

I'd pour my heart out to my mum about my weight anxiety and she would just be kind and reassure me that I looked fine. But the truth was I was fat because I ate too much. And the more miserable I felt about my weight, the more I would eat. When I was twelve, I started making my own way home from school and sitting about the house alone until my mum got in from work in the evening. I'd feel lonely and bored and fill my time with munching on whatever snacks I could find around the house: biscuits, crisps and large pint glasses of Nesquik flavoured milk mixed with ice cream. Sitting there stuffing my face with calories in front of Australian soap operas, I would try not to think about how this habit was getting out of control. My anxiety grew as my self-esteem plummeted.

The eighties were a brutal time. Body-shaming was not the taboo it is today. Even older relatives who should have known better seemed to revel in taking the piss out of me for my weight. I had to endure an evening at a family party where one of the older blokes got shitfaced and performed what could only be called a 'comedy roast' of me and my appearance for the entertainment of my brothers, who were also drunk. I was fourteen and had to sit there at his dining table while he bombarded me with machine-gun gags about how tubby I was. The harsher he became, the more my brothers howled and applauded, which encouraged him even more. I couldn't escape because I was fourteen and didn't have a car. When you're a kid, the dramatic walkout is not an option so you just have to sit there and take your medicine. That evening was hell and has lived with me for ever.

My father and all of his siblings (of which there were many as they came from Catholic stock) had done all right for themselves by this stage. They had grown up working class on a council estate but were all enjoying a period of success in the advertising industry – a sphere that was pretty meritocratic and was enjoying a particularly lucrative boom at the time. Their lifestyle seemed impossibly posh to me. Get togethers could be fun but sometimes felt alienating. I think Theo and Cas embraced it all; they went on to work in advertising and had no problem fitting in with the fancy-pants atmosphere.

Dom, like me, found it more uncomfortable. Dom was a postman with a shaven head and a couple of tattoos, way before body ink became run-of-the-mill. He didn't care about fitting in with people, especially not ones who seemed a bit snobby. This meant he would get the worst of it from some of our older relatives. They would mock him mercilessly for the way he spoke and looked, and I would get upset having to watch it happen. He and I felt a bit out of place among my dad's family sometimes. Sometimes, it looked to me a bit like bullying even if it wasn't meant that way. Dom was so messed up by these occasions that one time he nicked a bottle of vodka and locked himself in the toilet with it. When people finally realised he was missing they had to kick down the door, and they found the poor bastard lying passed out on the floor.

A relative once reprimanded me at a buffet for hacking at a piece of Brie in the wrong way. 'That's not the way we do it!' he guffawed as if I'd just taken a shit on the table. How was I supposed to know? We only had cheddar at my house and we usually grated it. It was only a small remark and he probably didn't mean to humiliate me, but I felt like a right cunt.

In another episode, a female relative screeched, 'Oh my God, Sam! You've got a double chin!' at me during a family barbecue when I was about eleven. I was all too aware of the state of my chin. She shouted the accusation loud enough for pretty much everyone else in the room to look round and stare. But she didn't stop there. 'I can't believe you've ACTUALLY got a double chin! How old are you now? How did it happen? This is terrible!' I've never been short of a quick, gobby response, not even back then. But it must have been a measure of how stung I was by her attack that I was only able to mutter 'Fuck off' at my own shoes and leave the room immediately.

My dad had kids really young and, while he tried to make it in rock 'n' roll and theatre, nothing ever took off. He was in his late thirties before he switched his attention to advertising which, back then, was a progressive industry where your background and qualifications didn't matter much as long as you had plenty of smart ideas. Between the sixties and eighties, the British advertising industry really took off thanks to an influx of clever people from largely working class backgrounds who managed to infiltrate it and shake things up through the power of their creativity (my dad and his brothers were part of the same generation as former admen like Alan Parker and the Scott brothers, Ridley and Tony). Things started to pick up for him when he got into writing ads because he was naturally funny, and smart by virtue of all the reading he'd done off his own back after leaving school at fifteen. His abilities with language had a huge impact on me: he has *savoir faire*, my dad. He always seemed to know what to say when we were out and about at weekends. He could be charming and funny. I learned from an early age the power of inserting the odd nifty phrase or expression into everyday chat: it seemed to get you noticed; sometimes it made people respect you more; often it made people laugh. I developed an ear for words and phrases that I found unusual or entertaining, and started to collect and memorise them. I wanted to be able to communicate like my dad. He also liked to live life well: good food, good music, good clothes – even when he was young and skint he'd try to have the best he could afford. I learned the importance of those everyday pleasures from him.

Sometimes my dad would help me with writing essays. He would get out these neat yellow pads of lined paper. Then he would take a sharpened pencil and write these beautiful, pithy, pin-sharp sentences in his impossibly attractive handwriting. Everything was always done 'straight into best' from the top of his head. He would take a point I'd scribbled down in three paragraphs and show me how to express it in just two dizzyingly concise lines. It wasn't just his use of words I wanted to emulate; it was the physical elegance with which he went through the process. I wanted to be like him. He showed me that my imagination wasn't just there for fun; it could be harnessed into something useful and appealing if I put enough effort into the execution.

From an early age, I took daft ideas extremely seriously. I came up with stupid sketches with my mates, conjured silly stories to make relatives laugh and once, in my penulti-mate year at school, co-wrote the school play, in which I also starred. I played a New York gangster who ran a speakeasy in the Prohibition era. Naturally, he had numerous girlfriends. The character's name? Sam Delaney. The name of the play? *Delaney's*. That's right, I wrote a school play in which I played a fantasy version of myself and named the whole thing after myself too. At least I tried to: the drama teachers cottoned on to the fact that my ego was getting a bit out of hand by this stage and insisted on changing the name of the play at the last minute, just before the official posters and tickets got sent to the printers. I was fucking fuming. I know I keep claiming that I was unsure of myself when I was a kid but my ego occasionally showed glimpses of the monster it would later become.

I've this brilliant auntie called Miki, who lived in Rome with my cousins, Alessandro and Daniele. I was really close to them. I absolutely loved it when they came to London and, occasionally, I would visit them in Rome. Miki had this boyfriend called Graham. He was a talented art director and photographer but was also really down to earth and unpretentious. He was from an ordinary background in Lancashire and, despite his success in the creative industries, was not in the least bit up himself. He was one of those adults who seem to be more interested in hanging out with kids than other grown-ups. He loved football, cricket and playing Subbuteo, and he was really funny. He spotted the fact that I had a big imagination and that I got a kick out of creating stuff. One day he found this homemade magazine I'd put together called the *Delaney Gazette*, which was just a bunch of stories I'd written about my family. I'd drawn pictures too and bound it all with staples. I hadn't really bothered showing it to anyone but he found it on a coffee table in my house and devoured it with such relish and delight. I was so proud and excited by his response.

He took me aside a few times after that to stress to me how important it was to make the most of my imagination and get even the daftest little ideas down on paper. He told me I had a talent for it and I had reason to believe him because he did that stuff for a living. But he wasn't talking to me about a career – he was stressing the simple joy that came from being creative. It didn't always matter if you made money from your ideas or even if other people paid attention. Just getting those ideas out of your head and making them real in some way was worthwhile in itself. It was fun and fulfilling. To this day, I can get such a big kick out of writing or drawing something just for my own entertainment.

When I visited my family in Rome, Graham would document the trip by drawing these hilarious cartoons of what we'd got up to each day. One day it was a caricature of me outside the Colosseum; the next it was a brilliant cartoon of me and my cousins watching Lazio play football at the Olympic Stadium. The only people getting a kick out of those cartoons were Graham, me and my cousins. They were little inside jokes that no one else would understand. When I got back home I stuck them all on my bedroom wall where they stayed for the next year. They weren't just a nice little memento of a great holiday; they were a reminder of the life-enriching joy of documenting the day-to-day in funny, silly, creative ways.

I was lucky to have met creative people at a young age. They were able to show me unconventional ways of living life and finding happiness. They pointed me towards a career in which I have been lucky enough to earn a wage out of creating stuff with words and pictures, first in magazines, then on radio and telly, and now in books and podcasts. I never take that for granted because I grew up in a house where my mum did jobs she mostly hated just to pay the bills. I lived in a street where all the neighbours got up and went to work in the dark doing tough work with their hands that paid them not much at all.

I was the first person in my family to go to university. My parents and my brothers had left school very early without much in the way of qualifications. But my brothers had worked hard to get their careers started – something I noted as I continued my academic studies into my early twenties. By the time I started work, my brothers had been grafting for over a decade and were doing really well for themselves despite their lack of qualifications. Dom started out as a postman at sixteen. Cas always had cool-sounding jobs from a young age like working in a clothes shop or being an usher at Hammersmith Odeon, where he got to watch loads of famous live bands for free. They were always hustling. Their example gave me a work ethic.

Theo, who had left school young and became a journalist before going on to make a tidy career out of directing commercials, also encouraged me to be creative; from a very young age, he'd make me really brilliant mix tapes, nurture my love of music and clothes, take me to the cinema to see cool films and – as I got older – encouraged me to think big about what I should do with my life. When I was still a student and his directing career was taking off, he looked after me. We'd go away on incredible boys' trips together to watch football matches in far flung places. He was ten years older than me but never treated me like a kid. I derived a huge amount of confidence from the way he treated me. We went to the World Cup in Los Angeles in 1994. He told me if I could sort my own plane ticket (which I did by working for six months in a call centre) he would pay for everything else. It was an incredible week. I could fill a whole chapter with the kind things Theo did for me when I was an insecure lad. Some were materially generous. As soon as he started to make a few quid, he started spending most of it on people he loved. One morning, on my twelfth birthday, I woke up and found a brand new Fred Perry next to my bed with a note saying he'd had to go to work early but had nipped round and left it as a gift on his way. What a bloke. It wasn't just the stuff he gave me though: it was the sense of friendship. He made me feel a bit special just by letting me hang around with him and by treating me as his equal. He laughed at my jokes and encouraged my endeavours. To have an older bloke like that in your life is an incredible boost to your confidence when you're still just a young whippersnapper. I felt liked by a bloke I admired. Slowly, that helped me to give less of a fuck about what other people thought of me.

It wasn't always easy, mind you. Kids were sometimes cruel about my weight too. That was to be expected. A pretty girl from the year above me invited me to a party once. I'd managed to make her laugh a few times at break time, which had got me noticed. I was only twelve and this was the first time I had received that sort of interest from a girl. I really fancied her and felt sure that the party would present an opportunity to nab my first kiss. But when I got there she was shitfaced on cider.

When I sidled up next to her on a bench and said 'Hello,' she looked me up and down and said, clear as a bell for every other fucker at the party to hear: 'Sorry, I won't kiss you because you're too fat.'

So. That was that conversation over with.

Incidents like that stung badly at the time, of course, but I was able to push them aside quite quickly and move on with life. Certainly, it was never enough to keep me indoors or turn me into an introvert. In fact, I was growing more confident and louder with each passing month – perhaps offsetting insecurities about my appearance by working on a big personality. I was able to make people laugh from a young age and didn't hesitate to launch into verbal confrontations either. There was a sliver of cruelty emerging in my own personality, which I probably nurtured to protect myself. I had a way with words and would often use this as a weapon against people, especially people I thought might be looking down on me.

The truth is, I had a chip on my shoulder. I don't think anyone tried to make me feel small. Some grown-ups I knew back then were so wrapped up in their own egos that they were careless and didn't stop to think about the collateral damage their behaviour was causing. As for the kids who said or did hurtful things, I think I realised even then that everyone was going through their own shit and that cruelty was often dished out by people who themselves felt insecure, unhappy or scared.

Again, I am hesitant to use the word trauma because it sounds so overblown. To be clear, I don't regard any of these childhood experiences I went through to be worse than the next person's. I know numerous people who went through much worse.

I'm repeating this but it's important for me to be clear: it is not the scale of your problems or traumas that matters as much as your ability to recognise them. I know that my experiences had an impact on who I became and how I felt about myself. I'm not saying they were catastrophic or insurmountable, but they definitely were relevant. By coming to understand that, I have been able to make better sense of my own feelings and behaviour. And, in turn, I have been able to find better ways of responding to life's challenges. I spent so long telling myself that nothing was wrong with me and that I had nothing to complain about. But I didn't have to complain about this stuff. I just had to recognise it for what it was: shit that had made me feel bad or scared or insecure when I was little and that had been living inside me ever since. I refused to see things that way for many decades, which meant that I was unable to understand all the things that eventually made my life unmanageable: the drinking, the drug abuse, the explosions of anger, the seemingly inexplicable periods of deep melancholy and the constant anxiety. I might not have had the worst life in the world, but comparisons – good or bad – are a waste of time. They can be destructive. I don't use any of the painful experiences of my childhood as excuses for my failings in adulthood. But by recognising the experiences and how they had an impact, I have at least been able to start processing them. And trying to get better. I'd advise anyone to have a crack at doing the same thing.

6

Tonight, I'm a Rock 'n' Roll Star

When I was fifteen years old I was visiting my cousin Daniele in Italy and, out of boredom, told him that I had formed an indie band in London that had become reasonably successful on the pub circuit.

Of course, there was no band – it was all complete fiction. A fiction I felt sure I could sell to him because (a) he lived in Rome and (b) there was no internet in 1990. How could he check my story? Anyone who was a fifteen-year-old boy in the pre-internet age will tell you that life was really boring back then and making up lies about yourself was one of the easiest and cheapest ways of passing the time.

I almost had my cousin convinced. Then he asked if I had any songs I could play him. Feeling cocky, I produced a C90 cassette and played him the song 'Freak Scene' by American alt-rockers Dinosaur Jr. The tape was sufficiently worn, and the recording sufficiently poor, for me to claim that it was me providing the lead vocals on the track. He listened carefully twice through, no doubt noticing the distinctive Massachusetts drawl of the band's singer J. Mascis and how it sounded nothing at all like my own reedy London squeak. Eventually, after some contemplation, he said: 'Fuck off, that's not you.'

What could I say? It was so very obvious that I had made up a stupid, transparent, pointless and pretty embarrassing lie. I couldn't just hunker down and stick to my story – it would make me look even more pathetic. But, I'm afraid, that's exactly what I did. I even feigned angry indignation that he didn't believe me. Things got pretty awkward between us. In the end, he just dropped the subject – out of what I presume was abject pity – and we never spoke of the matter ever again. Effectively, the lie still exists. Aged forty-seven, I have still not admitted to him that I am not, and never have been, the lead singer in an up-and-coming indie band. No wonder we don't talk as much as we used to.

It wasn't just boredom that had motivated my weird bullshit. It was also a desire to be respected. The need for respect runs pretty deep at that age, as you transition from the breezy life of being a child (children couldn't give a fuck about respect, they just want love and ice cream) into a frustrating state of semi-adulthood in which you want people to start taking you seriously (in spite of your shitty bum-fluff moustache and fantastical political views).

Wanting to be taken seriously can be really exhausting and destructive.

Exhausting because you go round acting like someone you're not. And destructive because you wind up thinking that the real version of yourself is not worthy of the respect you crave.

Although I grew out of telling such explicit lies about myself, I continued to adopt phoney personas well into adulthood. Like so many people, I wanted to seem cooler, tougher, more sophisticated and more resilient than I actually was. Appearing strong and resilient was a particular preoccupation. If someone said something mean I would never allow myself to show that I was hurt. If I was anxious or worried I could never let on, not even to myself. I adopted a right Jack the Biscuit persona, strutting about like I didn't have a care in the world. Worse, I sometimes acted like those people who did show emotions were pitiful and amusing to me. But when I went to bed at night, I had this mad habit of quietly muttering a little prayer in which I begged God not to allow any harm to come to me or my family. I must have got into that habit when I was about nine and I was still doing it in my twenties, while my girlfriend lay beside me. I dreaded the day she might hear my mutterings in the darkness.

'Sam, did you just say something?'

'Me? No.'

'Oh, sorry, I thought I just heard you pleading with God never to let you get cancer.'

'Hahahahaha. No. What? God? Cancer? Nope. That wasn't me. Definitely not the sort of thing I'd mutter. As you know, I don't believe in God. Anyway, night.'

A self-proclaimed atheist and cocksure superlad mumbling prayers under his duvet every night like the little Amish boy out of *Witness*? Fuck me, I was/am weird.

Like many people, I just couldn't allow anyone to think I was vulnerable.

Preaching resilience can sometimes sound like another way of saying 'suck it up' or 'deal with it'. It can be lazy and heartless – a way of belittling other people's feelings because you just can't be bothered engaging with them.

This is why we sometimes grow up to bullshit, lie and posture: because there is so much shame associated with having normal, human feelings. Emotions that have no connection with rational thought are natural. You can understand the science that keeps an airplane up in the sky but still be scared of flying. Feelings are weird, unpredictable and sometimes impossible to fully control.

So sometimes we feel sad or worried or sensitive or hurt even if there don't seem to be rational or obvious grounds for it. And out of shame we cover it up and contrive a resilience that, inside, isn't always there. We shrug and laugh stuff off. Why? Because we don't want people to judge us. Or to make it awkward for them. But fuck other people if they can't be bothered accepting the way you feel.

We just don't want people to know that we are human.

Which is a real shame because being human is what we're stuck with. And anyway, it's not all bad. It's better than being, say, a dog. Or a bumble bee – those poor fuckers sting people just once and immediately die, which must be gutting.

Anyway, here's my piece of life-changing advice: when you're feeling down, tell someone. And I don't necessarily mean tell someone in a serious 'I need a chat about my feelings' way (although that's a good idea too). I just mean get into the habit of being totally honest with everyone about what you might be going through. Get used to chucking it into conversation. You don't have to make people feel as if they are obliged to engage deeply with your feelings. Just let them know the feelings are there. Make it casual. Normalise being human.

Honour the way you feel: be open-hearted and honest, and you will feel so much better about yourself. You'll be surprised by the positive responses you get. It's also a handy way of filtering shitty people out of your life: those who mock or judge or belittle your feelings probably aren't worthy of your time.

Once, when I was about sixteen, I was mugged at Stamford Brook Underground Station by a gang of lads who pushed me and my mate Josh up against the wall on the staircase, roughed us up a bit, went through our pockets and took whatever change they could find. I'd been mugged before – it was not uncommon in my area back then – but this incident really shook me up. I went home to tell my older brother what had happened, hoping that he'd put together a posse of mates to go out and exact revenge. But he was drunk and belligerent and actually reprimanded me for allowing myself to get mugged. He called me soft. I told him I'd been outnumbered. He told me I should have been carrying a knife to protect myself. I went to bed and cried myself to sleep quietly.

The next night I cancelled the plans I'd made with mates. I told them I was feeling ill but the truth was I was badly shaken and couldn't face getting back on public transport. My mum bought me a four pack of Stellas to stay home with; despite me begging him not to, my brother had told her about the mugging. I guess the strong continental lager was her way of telling me she understood my pain.

By the time we were back at school on Monday, I'd turned the mugging into an amusing anecdote for my pals. That's what I always did. Getting mugged wasn't the problem as far as I was concerned; showing that I cared was what really scared me. Because I lived a mile or two from most of my mates, I often had to travel solo on my way home from nights out. I spent every journey on the bus or tube with my money hidden in my shoe, terrified that I'd get picked off by a gang. Sometimes I was and it was fucking horrible but I would always act to everyone else like it was water off a duck's back; just another pitfall of being young and adventurous and living in the city. But it was not water off a duck's back. It was fucking scary and horrible and it really did have an effect on me. Even in early adulthood, I couldn't walk down dark streets alone without checking over both shoulders constantly, hyper-aware of potential threats. It's not nice feeling on edge like that.

This was just another aspect of my youth that for years I chose to brush aside as I cultivated a carefree personality. 'Yeah, I got mugged once in a while – so what? Shit happens. Life is tough – but I'm tougher!' That was not only the persona I tried to project to everyone else – it was the one I started to actually believe was real. I convinced myself that none of these little moments of fear, sadness, pain or embarrassment had the slightest impact on me. You might wonder what good it does to dwell on this stuff anyway. Perhaps I was right to bury these incidents deep inside and avoid dwelling on them? Yes, I would agree that 'dwelling' sounds a bit too much like 'stewing' or 'fixating' on stuff – and not much good can ever come from that. Before you know it, you're so hung up on little things that happened to you in the past that you're unable to move forward. Worse, you can start to blame past problems for everything that's wrong with your present or even use them as an excuse for your failings.

That's not what I'm proposing. I try not to let the past hold me back. And I'm careful not to exaggerate the impact of these small incidents from my youth. I still have a good laugh retelling these anecdotes to my kids or reminiscing with mates. But I no longer deny the fact that they were painful as well as funny, and that they might have contributed to the way I felt or react to situations in adulthood. By identifying the roots of my hang ups I feel better able to unpick them. Or at least not judge myself so harshly for the way I am today. I look back at my younger self sometimes and think, *Fuck, that was really tough, I did well to get through that.* Which, if nothing else, makes a nice change from the usual self-criticism and trash-talk I subject myself to every day. We are all our own harshest critics.

And as someone once said: 'If someone spoke to you the way you spoke to yourself, you'd probably chin the bastard.' I agree.

The antidote to all this is a little bit of self-sympathy. It's different from self-pity. It starts with acknowledging the problems you faced at a formative age and the strength you showed to overcome them. And maybe giving yourself a quiet pat on the back once in a while for getting through the private pain that only you knew about.

7

How to Talk to Your Mates about Feelings and That

When I was seventeen, two of my best mates' mums died in quick succession. I had known both these lads, and their mums, since I was at nursery school. I had spent a huge portion of my childhood round their houses. In some ways their mums had been like spare mums of my own: cooking me tea, giving me lifts, sorting me out with plasters for my knees and that.

By the time we were seventeen we were part of a wider group of lads. Do you know how we all reacted when their mums died? We didn't. We just carried on without hardly mentioning it.

The first mum died close to Christmas.

I saw my mate, her son, the morning after it happened. We met up with the wider gang for a day of dicking about, going up town on the tube, smoking weed, playing pool, practising the elite-level time wasting that adolescent boys specialise in. He clearly just wanted to immerse himself in the numbing distraction of the usual routine. So when I saw him I mumbled: 'Sorry about your mum, mate.' And he looked down at his shoes and said: 'It's OK, cheers, yeah.' And that was that.

A few months later my other mate's mum died. He called me up one morning to tell me. 'Shit,' I said. 'You all right?'

'I'm OK,' he replied.

'Do you wanna come over to mine and watch a video?'

When he got there I had already put my copy of the Madness biopic *Take It or Leave It* in the VHS machine. But about forty minutes into watching it my mate said, apologetically: 'I'm not really enjoying this, can we watch something else?' The horrible sting of guilt still lives with me today. I knew he wasn't into Madness as much as I was. This was the worst day of his life. Why had I cajoled him into watching my own choice of film? I should have just said: 'Look, mate, your mum has just died. You choose the film.'

I suppose I could have told both of those friends about how deeply sorry I was.

I could have told them that I loved them and how I was there for them whenever they needed to talk. But the truth is, they would have hated that.

We'd grown up with an unspoken code: to never share our feelings. We liked football and lager and having dumb conversations about girls. And, you know, just being arseholes to each other. Being a Jack the Lad was about being carefree and brash; about taking the piss and never taking anything remotely seriously.

As I have already admitted, being a Jack the Lad is a right laugh. But it can also be dangerous. Because if your only way of dealing with bad feelings is to hide them behind bravado they will eventually consume you. Your only hope is that you never have any bad feelings. Good luck with that.

It doesn't have to be this way.

Being open about your vulnerabilities doesn't mean you have to give up on all the fun and laughter and shouting and beautifully mindless bollocks that you have built a large part of your personality around. You don't have to become the young Morrissey or the school counsellor out of *South Park* in order to start dealing with your feelings.

Men, particularly Jack the Lad types, need a more direct way of talking. The language that surrounds mental health can sound clinical and earnest and somehow excessively polite. Personally, I find it much easier to describe myself as being 'miserable', 'gutted' or 'having the right royal arsehole' than 'suffering from mental health issues'. It's hard to explain precisely why. Maybe it's because we don't feel comfortable with excessive sympathy. That we fear pity. That being made to feel like a victim or a sad case who needs to be somehow protected from scary words only serves to compound our feelings of worthlessness or anxiety or insecurity. Or maybe it's because 'suffering from mental health issues' just sounds like something a bit of a boring dickhead might say.

There is a big suicide problem among young men. This is not the time to be telling them to shape up and embrace the smug, middle-class lexicon of the wellness movement. Now is the time to find ways of making it easier for men to open up about their feelings in a way that comes more naturally to them.

We need to find a way of talking to our mates about this stuff that feels as natural as talking to them about football or telly.

Drop your mate a WhatsApp once in a while asking how he is.

He might try and fob you off with a standard: 'Yeah, fine.' But if you're worried he might be hiding something a bit darker, try and gently smoke it out. Try something like:

'Are you sure, you miserable cunt?' It might just start a more productive conversation.

I have some pals who are open to discussing this stuff. Hack, who I've known since I was eleven, has been through ups and downs with his mental health over the years just like me. We go for runs in Richmond Park together and talk through the shit that's bothering us or that we're worried about. We don't always offer each other solutions or advice; we help each other just by listening. To know that a mate understands, relates and sympathises is enough in itself. The first time Hack really opened up to me about his struggles was during a run by the river and, although I was gutted for him, I was delighted that he felt able to open up to me. I was honoured. And by telling him that I'd been through similar phases of worry, sleeplessness and self-doubt seemed to be a real help to him. Helping your mates feels incredible. Hack and I had grown up together so we spoke the same language, shared the same sense of humour and a similar worldview. So we were able to speak to each other in a language we both felt comfortable with. I remember him liking it when I described my anxiety as being in a state of 'constantly shitting myself'. It was just a small detail, a throwaway phrase, but that's the stuff that can make a difference: it can disarm a mate who might previously have been reluctant to engage in what they previously saw as psychobabble.

Hack does the same for me when I'm feeling miserable. He listens and understands but he is funny about it too. He makes me laugh while we talk about some of the darkest, deepest shit we've ever been through. It's during those chats, as we struggle through our runs, that I realise that to have a mate like Hack is a great privilege. When you're young you form bonds over pretty frivolous stuff like football, drink and drugs. But if you can stick together, and share all of the experiences that shape your personalities – the mad-lads holidays, the career struggles, the break ups, the births, the marriages and the deaths – you get a big reward later in life. That reward is someone who knows you almost better than anyone else and can talk and listen to you in a way that at times can feel life saving.

Not all of my closest mates are like Hack. Some aren't particularly keen to share at all. And that's fine. I try to look out for them in other ways by just staying in touch, checking in, making time to hang out, cheering them up with the sort of bullshit and banter we've always thrived on. Helping a mate through rough times doesn't have to involve deep and heavy conversations that last for hours. With some people, a lightness of touch is much better. To put it in the modern idiom, it's about making them feel 'seen'. It's about demonstrating you're interested in them, you're there for them and – whisper this bit because it's a fucking awkward thing for blokes to admit to their mates – you actually like them.

The truth is, I fucking love them. But, no, I would never, ever say that out loud. It would make them feel uncomfortable and that would be unfair.

We all get the hump with our mates sometimes. The older I get, the grumpier I am. Someone might piss me off with a throwaway remark when I'm in the wrong mood. But I try not to dwell on the negativity and remind myself that mates aren't your mates because they are perfect and never annoying. It runs deeper than that. They are your mates because you have a bond that was formed through years of dicking about together, getting drunk together, falling down together and getting back up together. Never underestimate the importance of the role your mates play in your life and never underestimate how important you are to theirs. Make an effort to stay in their lives, don't let things drift and make yourself available for either the most superficial or the most deep and meaningful chats, depending on their needs.

It's a shame we didn't see how important we were to each other when we were troubled teenagers in need of help. It would take us many more years and a lot more pain to start treating each other with the love and kindness we required.

8

That Time I Smoked Temple Balls and Had a Bunch of Eppies in Amsterdam

There's a lot of talk these days about self-care. It might sound a bit weird and hippyish but I'm a big fan, to be honest. Every Christmas I ask for blankets and candles because there is nothing I like better than cosying up on a cold winter's evening in front of the box, the soothing aroma of jasmine and lavender wafting out from melting wax, wrapped in something made out of cashmere, thinking about how lovely it is to just do fuck all once in a while.

Self-care is not that weird at all. Half the mental health problems I and most of my mates have struggled with in adulthood have been caused in no small part by the brutal and unforgiving nature of modern lifestyles. The 'work hard, play hard' culture that we all grew up around was ruinous for us. Long hours in unforgiving jobs followed by long nights in pubs and clubs, snorting powders, popping pills and drinking booze broke bits of our minds, our bodies and our souls. Throughout our twenties, life was lived at one hundred miles per hour against the backdrop of a permanent hangover. We never stopped to tell ourselves this was a mad and dangerous way to live because it's just how everyone seemed to live. We had no idea of what the alternatives were.

This had started when we were teenagers. Adventure and indulgence were our only agendas and taking care of ourselves was regarded as weak and pathetic. I was driving myself to the edge at a very young age and, despite plentiful warning signs, never really paused to imagine that I ought to slow down and take care.

'Hold up, lads!'

These were the last words I uttered before collapsing to the floor of the coffeeshop in Amsterdam. Bang! I went down like Apollo Creed in *Rocky IV*. My body erupted into a demented, jerking, foamy-mouthed seizure lasting three or four minutes. I knocked over tables and chairs, pissed my pants and ripped a fistful of hair out of my mate's head as he tried to restrain me. What a spectacle.

I was seventeen years old. Four mates and I were on an Interrailing trip around Europe. We were using stolen tickets that had been sold to us on the cheap by a bloke we knew from our local snooker club. The trip had been fun and stressful in equal measure. The drinking and adventure were great, but we were children really. We had hardly any money, even less common sense, knew nothing about where we were going, were hardly sleeping at all, were living off crisps and Coke and, it being 1992, we had no mobiles or other means of contacting home if we ran into trouble.

As I came around on that coffeeshop floor, drenched in my own urine, my vision blurred and my head pounding, I deduced that I had officially run into trouble.

'Temple balls gets them every time!' chuckled the proprietor as he rearranged all the furniture I'd knocked over. He was referring to the particularly strong strain of hashish my mates and I had been smoking just prior to my epileptic episode. He thought it was funny. He was the cunt who'd just sold it to us!

That was my first full-on epileptic fit. But I'd had minor episodes before that should have served as warning signs.

When I was twelve I had to undergo my 'cough-and-drop' with the school nurse. In case you don't know what a cough-and-drop is, it's a school procedure for twelve-year-old boys where they cup your ballbag and make you cough in order to check if your testicles have dropped yet. My older brothers, who had been through the same procedure years beforehand, delighted in winding me up about the prospect. 'The nurse grabs your bollocks and twists them really hard!' they warned. 'If you get a hard-on, don't worry, she keeps a metal spoon in a bowl of ice and whacks your knob with it at the first sign of trouble!'

As a result of these troubling stories, I arrived in the nurse's office on the big day riddled with anxiety. By the time she cupped my scrotum and asked me to cough, it had all got too much. My head started to spin and I collapsed.

When I came to, I was in the sickbay, where all poorly kids were held. As I lay prostrate on a camp bed in the corner, I noticed I had wet my pants. The next thing I noticed was Amy Wallace, a pretty and rather aloof girl from my year, sitting opposite me. I had never had the courage to speak with Amy before. Now, all sweaty and covered in my own wee, didn't seem like the most opportune moment. I tried a spluttering 'hello' but she just rolled her eyes.

Then the nurse came in and said: 'Oh you're awake, Sam! I'm afraid you passed out and wet yourself during your cough-and-drop – but don't worry we've called your mummy and she's coming to pick you up.'

For fuck's sake. I glanced again at Amy. She couldn't even bring herself to roll her eyes now. She just looked embarrassed for me.

When my mum arrived the nurse told her: 'When Sam was unconscious he started twitching on the floor in a peculiar manner. You should probably get him referred to a neurologist. Oh, and by the way, we also managed to establish that his left testicle is, as yet, undescended.'

We drove home in the rain, the piss drying slowly on my best school trousers as I peered silently out the window, wondering if Amy Wallace would ever consider dating an incontinent epileptic with one bollock. Can't lie, it was a shit day.

After the Amsterdam incident I was told by a specialist never to smoke marijuana or drink alcohol again, advice I completely ignored. I had several more fits in the years that followed, sometimes while drunk and high, sometimes not.

Looking back, I realise that all of my fits took place when I was in a state of high anxiety and stress. I don't think it was just the temple balls that wiped me out in Amsterdam. It was partly the unacknowledged stress of bumming round Europe with my mates when I was barely grown up enough to tie my own shoelaces. It felt wild being in the middle of faraway cities without any safety net and a sense that there was always trouble lurking round the corner. But we all just got on with it, had some fun and didn't allow ourselves to show each other any hint of fear or vulnerability.

Oh well, that's just part of being a teenage boy, I suppose.

At least it was in those days. If my son ever asks to go Interrailing for a few weeks using tickets bought from a man in a snooker club I will (even when he's twenty-seven, let alone seventeen) lock the dickhead in his room.

When I was fifteen, I was getting ready to go on my first proper date with my first proper girlfriend, Becky, when I collapsed in my mum's toilet and started twitching weirdly. The date was cancelled.

After completing twelve straight ten-hour shifts in a brand new job as a TV news reporter in my mid-twenties, I went home and suffered four consecutive seizures before being rushed to hospital in an ambulance and kept under observation for the weekend.

After West Ham beat Derby 5–1 in 1999, the day after my twenty-fourth birthday, I collapsed in a stranger's driveway on my way home, cutting my head open, having a fit and – you guessed it – pissing my pants again. That resulted in another weekend in hospital and six stitches in my nut.

These are just some of the highlights. Only recently have I come to realise that these incidents were caused by a refusal to take care of myself or acknowledge my own limits. But at the time I sort of laughed them off. After the initial physical and emotional shock wore off, I quickly turned them into entertaining anecdotes. But all those incidents were really fucking horrible. Coming round from a seizure is one of the most terrifying experiences I have ever endured. It's strange: people are talking to you, trying to help you regain consciousness, but it all seems otherworldly; you're floating above the room, unsure if you are alive or dead for about ten minutes. I feel sick just thinking about it.

Sometimes I wonder if those fits – some of them pretty massive – did any long-term physical damage to my brain.

I went for all the scans and stuff at the time, and they decided I was 'mildly' epileptic but that I didn't need medication. They predicted it would pass as I got older and that seems to have been the case. I haven't had a seizure since 2003.

The biggest learning I can draw from all of those messy incidents is that acknowledging my own stress is so important. So many blokes deny their stress to themselves and others: 'I'm fine . . . I'm not angry . . . I'm not stressed . . . I'm not tired . . . I AM NOT FUCKING SHOUTING!' We are so conditioned to hide vulnerability and maintain a stoic image that we don't even acknowledge to ourselves that we are feeling under pressure.

Once we do, it doesn't need to be a big deal. Rest when you can. Eat properly. Talk to someone, maybe. But the biggest and most important step of all is just admitting to yourself: 'Fuck, this is a bit scary.' Once you do that your body and mind can at least start to make sense of what the hell is happening.

9

It's Not that I'm Paranoid, It's Just that Everyone's Got It in for Me

I'll get on to talking to you about getting sober, going through recovery treatment and how I learned to better cope with my life in the second half of this book. For now, I will briefly tell you the first life-changing thing that a therapist ever told me: you cannot control the world.

This is both terrifying and liberating. Terrifying because it confirms your very worst fears that anything can happen at any moment, life is arbitrary and the world is a dangerous place. But it's liberating too because, once you accept your lack of control, you can chill out a bit and stop kidding yourself. There's a great deal of stuff you just can't account for so all you can do is shrug and deal with whatever is going on in the present.

This was a concept I had no understanding of when I was younger. I worked every day to try and secure a perfect life.

But it was not aspiration or ambition that drove me. I was fuelled by a constant hum of anxiety and also a pretty deep paranoia about the dark and malevolent forces that secretly conspired to trip me up at every turn. In big ways and small, I have been a right paranoid bastard my entire life. Some people might put this down to all the drugs I've taken but that's a bit trite, if you ask me. I was paranoid long before I tried my first spliff: I was always expecting the worst to happen. I thought people didn't like me and everyone was trying to stitch me up. The world seemed fake and perilous. Where did this come from? I'm not sure but it has caused me all sorts of trouble and misery over the years.

Sometime in the early noughties, when I was in my mid-twenties, I was in a nightclub in London with my girlfriend, my sister and a mate. We'd had a few drinks and were having a lovely time dancing to great music. Until, that is, I became suddenly convinced that a bunch of lads stood beside the dancefloor were pointing and laughing at us.

I don't know where this idea came from – it was probably the drink – but I started to fixate upon it so hard that I stopped having a lovely time and just disappeared inside my drunken, paranoid mind. And then, all of a sudden, I lunged at one of the lads, grabbed him by the throat and started to squeeze hard. He was understandably gobsmacked. Clearly, he hadn't even noticed my existence before I attacked him. The mockery had all been in my mind. I realised this quite quickly but, by that stage, I had taken things too far to back down. His mates tried to pull me off him and when that didn't work a couple of them rained a few punches at my head, which in turn drew my mate into the melee. Before we knew it, a fully fledged brawl had broken out.

102

Well, I say 'fully fledged'. It probably lasted about thirty seconds before the bouncers grabbed us and threw us on the street. I recall one of them clutching my face in his hand and saying with a sort of urgent compassion: 'What are you doing, mate?'

It was a fair question. I didn't know the answer. Nor did the lads I had attacked or my mate who had nobly stood up for me and taken a couple of digs for his troubles. My girlfriend and sister were completely befuddled and a little outraged. I ended up saying sorry to the lad I'd tried to strangle as I stumbled away from the scene. He accepted the apology with an expression that seemed to say: *You wanna get your head checked, you fucking weirdo.* He was right, of course.

In the morning I woke up hung over, full of regret but happy to write the whole thing off to pissed-up misadventure. Just one of those things, no harm done, maybe try to pace myself a bit better next time I'm out.

But there was more to it than that. I was a paranoid person, I just didn't realise it. Throughout my teens, twenties and thirties I thought that everybody was out to get me.

If a stranger was sniggering in a public place, I often assumed they were sniggering at me. At work, if a couple of colleagues were having a meeting behind closed doors, I automatically assumed they were plotting my professional downfall. In my relationship, I was jealous and suspicious a lot of the time for no good reason whatsoever. I couldn't quite accept that my girlfriend really loved me, or even liked me, that much. For years, I suspected that our relationship was a scam she was carrying out while she looked for someone better. It can't have been much fun for her.

All this paranoia was exhausting. The attempted nightclub strangling was a one off – I've never really been a violent person. Mostly I kept all the rage and suspicion inside, desperate to show that I didn't care that *every bastard was trying to stitch me up.*

It's pretty likely that the unpredictable nature of my childhood played a big role in cultivating all of this paranoia. As a kid, you put blind faith in your parents. But because your parents are human beings – and not the deities you believe them to be – they inevitably let you down sometimes. My dad left us; my mum was prone to bringing home new boyfriends or inviting strange friends to kip down on our sofa for months on end. She didn't like confrontation and had a tendency to say whatever was needed to make me feel better when I was anxious or upset. Even if that thing wasn't strictly true. She did this not out of malice or weakness but out of love. I never blame her for any of this stuff because the fact that she managed to raise the four of us with so much love and kindness without descending into complete mental collapse or addiction is beyond my comprehension. I fell into addiction when I had just two kids, a nice house, a good career and a stable, loving marriage. So, to me, my mum is a fucking superhero. But, the fact is, I never felt as if I could completely rely on the words or actions of the significant adults in my life and that might have been where my paranoia stemmed from.

Plus there was this: one afternoon when I was twenty years old my mum revealed that I had an older sister that she had never told me about. My parents had her when they were very young and, under pressure from their parents, opted to have the baby adopted. They subsequently stayed together and, later, had my brothers and me. For whatever reason, neither my mum nor dad had ever told me about her. I don't resent either of them for this: they had their reasons. It was all very traumatic for them and if they felt unable to discuss it then I understood. Nevertheless, the realisation, aged twenty, that a secret of that magnitude could have been kept from me my entire life was pretty shocking. It turned out that literally everyone else in my entire extended family had known about this sister for years: my brothers, my brothers' wives, my uncles, my aunts, my cousins, even their pals who I'd never met. Literally every fucker knew about my sister other than me. I wasn't angry, I was amazed. I was rather impressed by the grand scale of this conspiracy of silence.

To cut a long story short, my sister, Annie, later became a part of my life and we have formed what I regard as a really special bond. She is an amazing sister, a beautiful person and a brilliant presence in my life. I am extremely lucky to have her. Plus, after the years and years in which my mum secretly tortured herself over what might have happened to the daughter she gave up, I am delighted that they eventually reunited and put some of those ghosts to rest. All's well that ends well – and I regard the story of my sister, my parents and my family to be a real-life fairy tale with a beautiful ending.

Having said all of that, the whole episode sent my already twisted and paranoid brain over the edge. I mean, if everyone I loved and trusted could keep a secret that big from me for that many years then could I really believe anything I saw or heard ever again? Not really. I developed major trust issues. I simply couldn't have 100 per cent faith in anyone ever again. It was horrible for the people around me but, for what it's worth, it was fucking horrible for me too.

I am still not over this completely but I have learned, mostly through therapy, to just ignore my own thoughts sometimes. When paranoia starts to bother me, I watch it from a distance and remind myself that these thoughts aren't rational. They are just a trick my brain is playing on me. A trick that stems back to experiences I had when I was younger. And that those experiences don't have to shape my perception of everything that happens to me in the present or future.

For years, I resisted analysing any of my irrational behaviour because I was ashamed of what I might discover. A lot of people worry that admitting to mental illness might make them seem weak. But my biggest fear was that it would make me seem stupid. I had been brought up to think that emotional struggles were the result of intellectual shortcomings. I thought that if I felt irrationally sad, angry, worried or afraid it was just that I lacked the intelligence to properly understand a situation. So if I did something dumb or irrational, I was quick to dismiss it as a daft anomaly that wasn't in any way reflective of my true personality.

But I have come to realise that the best form of intelligence is the ability to see how unintelligent I am capable of being. Once you know you're liable to think daft thoughts or act in dumb ways, you've got a much better chance of controlling yourself.

The brain is unreliable. It sends us dodgy readings and bullshit guidance every day.

Socrates boiled all of philosophy down to one line: 'Know thyself.'

We can be fucking stupid. To accept that means that we can mitigate against our most destructive thoughts and actions. Self-reflection is not a sign of stupidity; it is perhaps the most valuable expression of human intelligence.

10

How to Drown in Your Own Life

I don't know if you've ever been to Disneyland Paris but, if you have, you will understand why it is one of the worst places in the world to have a miscarriage. You're surrounded by actors dressed up in princess outfits exuding contrived gleefulness. The wallpaper in the hotel is covered in illustrations of *Bambi* and *Dumbo*. Barmy, saccharine soundtracks from *Beauty and the Beast* and *The Little Mermaid* pump hauntingly from speakers wherever you go. The inescapable ambience of synthetic joy is suffocating. It's no place to experience landmark trauma. They're just not set up for it.

And I write as someone who happens to love Disney. The animations, the stories, the songs – I can't get enough. Actually, that's not true. I can get enough. In 2010, when my wife miscarried in the bathroom of our room at the Disneyland hotel, with my daughter and two young nieces sleeping in the next room, I discovered how much Disney was enough Disney for me.

* * *

We had been trying for a second child for over a year. When nothing happened after six months we went to see a private specialist on Harley Street. I jumped in a cab one lunchtime and rushed across town from my office to an expensive fertility clinic, where I was booked in to have a wank into a cup. I had scanned the instructions they had emailed me in advance and they had mentioned that I should not ejaculate for a couple of days in advance, in order to maximise my output. I had been quite diligent in observing this – I doubled down for extra safety and took care not to let anything out of my ballbag for a whole four days in advance. I figured the more they had to work with in the lab, the better. When I arrived slightly late and harassed at the clinic they asked me when was the last time I had ejaculated and I told them proudly that it had been a whole ninety-six hours. But I didn't get the applause I was expecting.

'Oh dear, that's too long,' the nurse said, frowning.

'But I thought I was supposed to save it up?'

'Yes, Mr Delaney. But not for four days – there will be dead sperm in there now.'

Great. I had wasted a whole lunchbreak on a futile and expensive taxi ride to a wank bank that wouldn't let me make a deposit. And I was backed up with dead sperm. Miserable and frustrated, I called my wife and apologised for my miscalculations, promising to return for another go in two days' time.

Trying for a baby is not always as magical and romantic as movies lead you to believe.

We went through various appointments with a variety of doctors during that period – baffled as to why we weren't able to make a baby. We'd managed to have one before, so clearly our bodies were capable in a mechanical sense. What had changed?

'You're working too hard,' said my gran when I went to visit her in the care home one day. She was in her late eighties, a mum to eight children, grandma to dozens of grandchildren and great-gran to a few more. I suppose that qualified her to give a bit of advice on reproductive matters, but that's not the way I saw it at the time.

'Thanks, Gran, but I don't think work has got anything to do with it. Busy people get pregnant all the time.'

As it turned out, I think she was right – and listening to her might have saved me a great deal of time, money and stress.

My wife and I were in our mid-thirties and taking adulthood really seriously. We had sold up in Notting Hill, bought a cottage in leafy, suburban Barnes, enrolled our daughter in the local nursery and bought a sensible car. We'd thrown ourselves into this shit. We wanted a sibling for our daughter for sincere reasons. We were driven by love. But people ask you all the time when you're that age about your plans for procreation, like it's as much their business as your summer holiday plans. Having a second kid fitted a prescriptive, middle-class lifestyle template that, try as we might, we were being hoodwinked into following. I'm not saying that a second child was a phoney lifestyle choice; but the fact that we were in a hurry about it – frantically trying to fit it into our lives between demanding careers, exhausting commutes, childcare, perpetual lack of sleep, caffeine addiction and the weekend partying that we, like many first-time parents, thought it was perfectly possible to maintain to pre-parenting levels – was our problem. I can see that now. It was probably what my gran was getting at.

Eventually, Anna got pregnant, and we were euphoric. Not content with the money wasted at the over-picky sperm clinics, we chucked more money at the situation by hiring a private obstetrician who would guide us personally through pregnancy with regular scans, bits of advice and calming chats in his well-appointed consultancy room.

Were we stupid? Yes. We had been driven that way by anxiety. We had a sense of urgency about this second child that was not healthy for either of us, either mentally or physically.

What difference will a private obstetrician make when you're in Disneyland Paris on a hot Saturday night in May listening to your wife sob in the bathroom because she has started to bleed? That's just her body rejecting the pregnancy. You can't pay your way out of it. You just call reception and, after sitting on hold while the voice of Goofy sings at you, ask them if they can arrange for a doctor to come to your room. A real one, please, not someone in a Mickey Mouse outfit wearing a stethoscope round their neck.

I went into the adjoining room to check on the kids. I told them that Anna was feeling poorly and had to see the doctor. It was pretty late in the evening so they were slightly suspicious but the good thing about kids in a crisis is that they generally don't give a fuck as long as you let them watch TV and give them something to eat.

The doctor briefly examined Anna in our room and sent for an ambulance. I couldn't accompany her to the hospital because I had to stay with the kids. She endured a cold, miserable and lonely examination at the hands of an indifferent doctor who eventually told her, in the most casual of terms, that the baby was 'gone'. She got back to the hotel at one in the morning and we both held each other and cried.

I cut the trip short, made up a lie to the kids and booked a train to take us home the next morning. They were gutted. The journey home was silent. We were heartbroken.

* * *

At the end of that year I left my job. We still hadn't managed to get pregnant again. Life seemed to be in limbo. I was strung out, exhausted and unhappy. On the face of it, being offered the job as editor of *Heat* magazine eighteen months previously had been a godsend. It was a famous and successful magazine, and the job was one of the most sought after in the industry. It came with a whopping salary too. I'd been struggling to complete a book (I can't even remember what it was about) and doing bits of freelance work. I'd also been taking care of my daughter after my wife had returned to her demanding job in the West End. I had been feeling a bit directionless and bored, and the world had suffered a financial crash just a matter of months beforehand. There were genuine fears that we all might end up destitute and homeless, so when the job offer came completely out of the blue it felt like the answer to everything. To be offered a high-flying job with a contract and all the other benefits that went with it was incredible; it was too much to turn down. As my wife said to me at the time: 'You'd have to be some sort of wanker not to take it.'

But there was one problem with this job: I didn't want to do it. Deep down inside, I knew it wasn't for me. It was celebrity gossip. I enjoyed reading it, sure, but I had never dealt in it professionally and I didn't care enough about it. A job like that demands a huge amount of time and energy – the sort of time and energy I can only really fuel with passion. But I didn't feel any passion. So I would just have to run on fumes.

Expecting every job to fulfil you in some meaningful, spiritual way sounds a bit fucking entitled, I admit. Turning down a ton of money to edit an iconic magazine would have been arrogant and spoiled of me, I suppose. At least that was what I told myself at the time. I didn't want to look a gift horse in the mouth: that wasn't who I was.

I completely switched off from what my heart was telling me. This was part of a pattern that controlled my life for a long time: thinking too much about perceptions and not enough about what I actually wanted to do. I'd never grown out of it. I created an ideal for myself – based largely on what I thought other people might expect or approve of – and held myself to that standard mercilessly. I beat myself up constantly for not conforming to an artificial ideal. Becoming a magazine editor was something to which I'd always aspired. I was obsessed with magazines from an early age. I loved the humour, the writing, the beautifully designed pages – even the touch and smell of them drove me wild. I started out reading *Look-in* when I was a kid before graduating to *Smash Hits*, the *Face* and eventually *Loaded* when it first came out. They were all like portals into an exciting world I couldn't otherwise access. By the time I was a politics undergraduate at Sussex University, my only ambition was to get involved in the then thriving magazine industry.

So when I finally worked my way up far enough to be offered the top job at one of the top mags in the country, I couldn't say no. I didn't stop to think hard enough about whether it was the right fit.

I took that mad job at a massive magazine with demanding bosses and a large staff. It was fun – of course it was – but it was relentless and unforgiving, and I felt completely out of place from day one. I didn't allow myself to admit that to anyone at the time and I didn't really admit it until now because I was too scared of sounding entitled. I know what it's like to do shit jobs just to make ends meet. My mum was often ill, occasionally depressed, always stressed, but she did them because she had rent to pay and mouths to feed. And there are millions of others who expect nothing more than that from life. Who was I to expect that a job would not only be fun, well paid and glamorous, but also deeply nourishing to me on an intellectual and spiritual level?

But do you know what? I was right to expect more. I was wrong to beat myself up for feeling unhappy in that job. There was nothing wrong with the *Heat* job. It was a great job. It just wasn't the right job for me. I should have listened to my heart in the first place and never taken it. I wasn't living a life that was true to myself – that matched my true feelings and desires faithfully. That is at the heart of much pain and dissatisfaction in our lives, I reckon. We are surrounded by so many messages about how to live or what represents success that we lose sight of what we want or need personally. It leads to a sort of spiritual and mental confusion where you are living life against your own instincts.

It's so easy to fall completely deaf to your own better instincts because you are so busy trying to live an artificial version of yourself that you think might impress others. And then you wonder why you're always sad and stressed despite everything seemingly going so well. You drink and take drugs to numb those dark feeling of disconnection and discomfort. They are really scary because you can't even see where they are coming from. As I would later find out, drink and drugs can really help sweep them away at times.

When I left my job at *Heat* I was able to relax a bit more. I went for walks in the middle of the day. I sat outside and watched the geese swimming on the pond. I visited my mum, had the odd lunch with my dad, caught up with mates, listened to music on the radio. I picked my daughter up from nursery and took her to the swings and slides on sunny afternoons. For a while, it seemed like I was really on a path to finding myself again. To discovering the stuff that really made me happy and forgetting all of the noise and nonsense that had led me down the wrong paths in the past.

And then Anna became pregnant again. We were nervous that she might lose another baby. Three months passed, then six months. We went in and out of the hospital (we had seen sense and given up all the private bollocks by now), getting scans that told us this baby was real and healthy and very much on its way into our lives. We took our daughter Coco to the pub one afternoon and told her she was going to have a little brother or sister. She was so happy and excited. It was a beautiful moment. Everything had worked out for the best. I thought about what my grandma had said about working too hard and it finally made sense. It hadn't just been that I was physically knackered; I was mentally and emotionally exhausted too. All it took was a few months of getting back to the real me for all the stress, anxiety and self-doubt to melt away. Now the baby was on its way and life would unfold just the way we had been hoping.

For the next few weeks I felt better than I had done in years: relieved, relaxed and ready for where this next chapter might take me. But then, suddenly and without warning, I started waking up in the night in a state of complete panic. Each night it happened earlier and earlier until eventually I hit the point where I wasn't getting to sleep at all. The moment my wife nodded off, the silence and darkness would envelop me and a tornado of troubling thoughts would start spinning around my head.

My mind fixated over anything and everything: money, work, relationship, health, mates, family. My brain was exhausted and vulnerable – just like your body is susceptible to injury when you are physically exhausted. I obsessed constantly over the most trivial of concerns. I felt unable to break the constant cycle of worry.

The moment my wife woke up in the morning I would start rabbiting at her about all of these crazy, inconsequential issues as if they were the end of the world. She was already coping with the physical, hormonal and emotional stress of pregnancy plus the exhausting, day-to-day pressures of work and, rather than helping her get through it all, I was compounding problems with my own insanity. I was at least self-aware enough to label my behaviour as a type of insanity. I understood that my feelings weren't entirely rational but, nevertheless, I couldn't stop them. When my wife went to work, I felt alone and consumed by dread about every last trivial problem in my life. Plus I continuously projected future problems, speculating wildly about worst-case scenarios and convincing myself that they were inevitable. I was terrified of the future and lost faith in my ability to provide the stability and comforts my family would need.

If anyone tried to help by explaining why all of these fears were unlikely to ever be realised, I could listen, I could agree and I could understand: but it would make no difference whatsoever to the way I felt.

At that stage, I don't think any appeal to the rational parts of my mind could have helped. I look back and realise that I was in a state of complete burnout. I needed a bit more self-awareness about my problems. I needed to recognise when I was feeling stressed and appreciate the need to do something about it. Had I been able to do so, I could have dealt with them at an early stage. I could have given myself the compassion and rest I needed along the way. Not big, radical lifestyle interventions like rehab, but the little things that help you balance life out. The ability to say 'no' to superfluous work or social engagements from time to time. The will to take time out from everything, just for an afternoon, and surround yourself in peace. Read a book, go for a walk, stare out the window for a while. Release myself from the constant self-imposed pressure to be moving forward. I thought all that stuff was bollocks: it was for people who were weak and scared. I thought I was special, that I had a superhuman ability to cope with more pressure than the average bloke. To be more productive. I secretly judged my peers for being a bit lazy. Being lazy was one of my biggest fears. I wanted to be relentless. That, I believed, was the secret of my success so far.

I was wrong about everything.

Being relentless is the worst possible aspiration you can have in life. I had been riding a train destined for burnout since I was in my early twenties. The warning signs had been there along the way: the periods of sadness that I would try to ignore and drink away; the daily, low-level hum of anxiety that I would distract myself from with more work; the state of agitation and insecurity that I would channel into ever wilder plans and ambitions; the seizures; the occasional explosion of temper or act of childish petulance.

I kept going: trying to work harder, trying to achieve more and hoping that, eventually, I would arrive at a place of complete contentment where every problem in my life had been eradicated. By what? I wasn't sure. Money and status, probably. I assumed that I would achieve a position in life that would somehow incubate me from all the things that scared me, like failure, loneliness, ill health, poverty, ridicule, boredom.

But no matter how hard I worked, no matter how carefully I schemed and no matter how fast I went, I never seemed to get any closer to that state of contentment. In fact, the harder I tried, the worse I felt. I was trying to swim against a current that dragged me down harder the more I struggled against it. My frustrations grew stronger, often manifesting themselves as anger and bitterness. Drink and drugs were always the easiest remedy.

Meanwhile, I had so much. I had a loving relationship; I had a home; I had friends and relatives I cared about and with whom I loved spending time; and I enjoyed the work I did. I had everything going for me – I had so many advantages in life. And, believe me, I was aware of all of this. I wasn't blind to all the good stuff in my life. I knew I was lucky and so I felt deeply ashamed of feeling sad. It was a massive secret. Such a big secret that I threw everything into appearing happy and carefree. I reacted to periods of sadness and worry by acting out a hyper-positive, hyper-confident persona. I was really good at it. But it was fucking exhausting and only compounded the stress I was under.

Let's be clear: all of the stress was self-manufactured. This had started before I had kids and a mortgage. As I have described, I had been plagued by fear and anxiety since I was a kid. I had never been able to get rid of it because I kept it secret. I assumed I was the only person in the world with feelings like these.

When you're a young man, living out loud with your mates in the pub every night, anxiety is not a good look. It is the antithesis of the image you are trying to project. Nobody wants to hear about the dark moments and praying to yourself in your room at night. It is, objectively, fucking weird. And so you carry around the secret about your nervous-ninny alter-ego and the whole thing gets worse and worse.

I even used to hide it from my girlfriend when we first got together because I figured that being angsty was a stone-cold turn off to women. I assumed (wrongly, of course) that Anna had been attracted to me because of my swaggering barroom confidence, bawdy humour and Jack the Lad charisma. I was too scared to reveal the other side of me that secretly shat himself that he was going to get ill or fail in life or be discovered as a fraud with a sensitive soul. These assumptions were a real disservice to Anna, who never showed me anything but unconditional love and understanding and, besides, she is far too smart and imaginative to have ever been impressed by the superlad side of my personality. It took years for me to understand that she had fallen in love with me in spite of my laddish tendencies, not because of them. Young men are really stupid, and I was no exception. I sometimes can't believe that she stuck with me for so long, waiting for me to figure this stuff out for myself.

When I talk about stress and exhaustion, I don't mean the sort you see executives in old movies suffering from. I wasn't wrapped up in suffocating corporate slavery; neither was I struggling in poverty. I had a fairly average amount of ordinary concerns and preoccupations. For most of my adult life, I used drugs and alcohol to manage my moods but no more than many of my peers. The problem, all along, was inside me. I was the one putting myself under extra pressure to project a certain personality. I was the one obsessing over professional success. I was the one judging myself harshly for being unproductive. And I was the one constantly nurturing fear about the future. Why? Perhaps something was missing. Perhaps there was a void inside that made me feel the real me was never good enough.

Maybe this was compounded by a culture that seemed to encourage and provoke all of my worst insecurities. Especially when I was coming of age in the 1990s, the era of laddism, *Loaded* and Britpop, acting the dickhead was actually celebrated. Look at Liam Gallagher, the crown prince of nineties lad culture, getting up on stage at the 1996 Brit Awards, totally off his nut, wearing a big sheepskin coat, John Lennon glasses and a mad, death-throes Jim Morrison beard. Swearing, shouting, abusing everyone in the audience and then pretending to bum himself with the auspicious industry award he'd just been handed. I remember watching that with a bunch of mates in a dingy student house in Brighton and laughing my head off. He embodied the worldview we all subscribed to: a fuck-you nihilism perfectly described in his brother Noel's lyrics about embracing the sunshine, doing the white line and living like a rock 'n' roll star. The generation before us, who had come of age in the eighties, had seemed like an earnest bunch: forever on student marches in their big overcoats, moaning about Thatcher, the miners or nuclear bombs. My generation started drinking just after the Berlin Wall came down and people started organising massive raves in fields; our theory was that nothing can touch you as long as you take nothing seriously. Nothing is real, everything is bollocks, so just get on with giving it large and everything should turn out fine.

Unfortunately, our inner lives are inescapably more complex than that. As appealing as it sounded, getting pissed all the time, watching lots of football and avoiding any contemplation of our feelings was never going to be a practical design for life.

The problem with adulthood is that it just happens all around you without your control. A series of events can unfold so rapidly that it can sometimes feel that you are just a passenger on a train that is being driven by unknown forces. You leave school or university, you get a job, you start a relationship, you get yourself a home, get married, have kids. Everything seems like it's jogging along as it should be. You have no reason to think that anything is wrong because, externally, everything looks in order. But how much have you changed internally? How ready are you to deal with the rapid change in circumstances, the increased responsibility, the new pressures and expectations? Without getting your head around this stuff, discussing it with other people, developing the self-awareness and sense of perspective you need, it can feel like you're a helpless cork on the ocean. You smile through it all, giving everyone the impression that you're in total control because to open up and say, 'Lads, I just can't handle this crap – I feel like I'm fucking drowning' is embarrassing. Why is it so embarrassing? Because everyone else you know is working hard to give off the impression that they're in complete control too. We are all playacting that life is easy and we're OK. By doing this we are contributing to each other's sense of isolation and fear.

I grew up believing I could talk to my three brothers about anything and that they could do the same with me. But there is an unspoken competitiveness among all siblings, especially brothers. None of you wants to look like you're falling behind the others. None of you wants to admit to a weakness that the others don't show. Yes, I could go to my brothers with something that we would all deem to be a 'big deal' – like a break up, or the loss of a job, or a health issue. But could I go to them and just admit that the very basics of life – being a dad, paying the bills, navigating a marriage, managing a career – were swallowing me up? That I was drowning in what was, on the face of it, a pretty ordinary life not dissimilar to the ones they were living? No. I don't think any of us would have made that admission to each other. It would be too easy to have taken the piss. If one of my brothers had made that sort of confession to me, hand on heart, I might have scoffed. I might have said something sarcastic like: 'Oh dear me, the mortgage on your nice big house is troubling you, is it? My heart bleeds.' Such is the nature of brotherly relationships. But it's not just brothers being arseholes to each other. There is a culture of judgement that is thriving everywhere today. No one is safe admitting to any vulnerability because there will always be someone on social media waiting to point out all the people who have it much, much worse than you.

The whole point of this book – and all of the brilliantly open conversations that people are sharing these days – is that mental health problems are something everyone has; that we all have complex and confusing feelings that we have to cope with every day. Material circumstances cannot change that. It's about being human.

I don't doubt that the King has off days. I'd be surprised if Jeff Bezos doesn't sometimes wake up in the night with the raging hump about some snide comment a mate made over dinner ten years previously. I don't for a minute presume that wealth, class or privilege incubate you from the natural ebb and flow of your mental health.

Years ago, I remember hearing about a professional footballer who had received treatment for mental illness; his manager at the time actually laughed about it in a press conference, calling into question how someone on such a high wage could possibly be depressed. It was a jaw-dropping moment that people sometimes use to illustrate how far we have come in our attitudes to mental health. Because, these days, no one would suggest that money protected anyone from depression, right? Wrong.

In many respects we are more divided than ever. Every day, social media and the newspapers are filled with people judging others. The crux of that judgement is very often based around their right to feel the way they do. How dare that person say that? How could they possibly understand the realities of life?

We are often calling into question people's right to feel the way they do.

I don't like Boris Johnson and I think he was an awful prime minister. But in 2021 I read that his mum had died. This was reported in the press as a passing, almost inconsequential news story. The prevailing attitude seemed to be: *Boris Johnson is the prime minister; he is rich; he went to Eton; he has fucked up the country, so fuck him.* I might have even allowed myself to think those exact thoughts. But Boris Johnson is (and I can't believe I am saying this – but I have chosen the most extreme example I could think of in order to really nail my point here) a human being, just like you and me. He felt the same feelings about his mother as any other human being does. And we have no reason to believe that his sense of crushing sadness would have been any less than the next bereaved son. He should have been given a month off, at the very least.

Mental health has become caught in the crossfire of the culture wars. But if we are serious about treating mental health with the same degree of seriousness as we do physical health, then we really have to take context out of it. The point is: we are all fucked up. If we really want to start helping each other, we need to start taking everyone's pain seriously.

11

Here Comes the Fear Again

My cousin's wedding in Tuscany in 2010 was supposed to be an idyllic family weekend full of love, laughter and good times. And it would have been had I not received a letter from the Inland Revenue the night before I left and gone absolutely batshit crazy.

I was thirty-five and still the editor of *Heat* magazine. I was well paid, had a secure contract, owned my own house and was married with a two-year-old daughter. Everything in life was going great. But the night before we were set to fly out to Italy, I found a brown envelope on the doormat emblazoned with the chilling letters 'HMRC'.

My heart leaped up into my mouth.

Why? My tax affairs were as dreary and straightforward as the next dickhead's. I was hardly stashing millions in the Cayman Islands or investing in dodgy movie projects like all those tax-swerving celebs you hear about. I had nothing to hide. But I was a neurotic when it came to anything to do with money or admin.

More than that, I had a scary belief in arbitrary karma. I believed that the universe was programmed to punish excessive happiness with occasional bouts of intense sadness.

My mind buzzed with this irrational narrative, whereby any lengthy period of good fortune would have to be counterbalanced at some point by a huge dose of bad luck. I claimed to be a devout atheist – I thought that made me sound clever – but, in fact, I secretly believed in the existence of a sadistic God who occasionally punished you for being happy by chucking a bucket of shit on your head.

So, whenever life seemed good, I was always on the lookout for something bad to happen.

The letter inside the brown envelope informed me that my accountant was under investigation for some sort of iffy practices. I didn't really understand what the accusations were; in fact, I didn't finish reading beyond the first paragraph. If I had, I would have realised that I personally was under no scrutiny whatsoever and that this letter – sent out in identical form to the accountant's hundreds of other clients – was just a courtesy heads-up from the Revenue.

But the words 'your accountant' and 'investigation' were enough to send me into a mental tailspin. Within ten minutes I was calling everyone else I knew who used the same accountant to compare notes and strategise a collective legal defence. It being a Friday night in August, they were all either on holiday or out having fun – not sitting at home working themselves into a frenzy over an imaginary scenario in which they would have to sell their homes to avoid white-collar prison.

But that was exactly what I was doing. I managed to get a friend's husband on the blower – a barrister – to discuss the situation. He was a good bloke who politely attempted to allay my fears. But, at the end of the day, he was a barrister used to

124

defending violent criminals in court. Not a tax lawyer, much less an accountant. He should have just laughed and told me I was mental. It would have helped.

My wife, the only person who had stood between me, my constant irrational worries and a full nervous breakdown for the previous ten years, tried her best to contain my sudden meltdown.

She says now that it was the worst she had ever seen me. I was frantic, pacing the living-room floor with the letter clutched in my fist, rambling about receipts and invoices and bookkeepers and legal teams and the cell conditions at Ford Open Prison.

None of this is an exaggeration. It is the only time I have seen the intensity of my anxious ravings penetrate my wife's zen-like rationality. She ended up crying that night out of frustration and fear. But that was just the start.

The next morning, having not slept the entire night, we arrived at Gatwick departures with me speaking at a hundred miles per hour down the phone to an understandably bewildered accountant – the friend of a friend – who I had never met but had managed to contact at home on a Saturday morning in order to seek a second opinion.

On the plane, I was still pressing the mobile to my ear, demanding reassurances from this poor bastard while my wife and various flight attendants ordered me to end the call because we were about to taxi.

Once in Tuscany, at the old farmhouse where everyone was staying, I was greeted by dozens of relatives – many of whom I hadn't seen for years. It was sunny and beautiful. But I was absolutely bananas. Theo arrived in high spirits with his wife and children, and I immediately collared him, dragging him into a side room to pour out my batshit theories about the accountant, what he had been up to and how it was going to land me destitute, imprisoned or quite possibly both.

Because Theo is a nice bloke, he, just like everyone else I had subjected to this line of mad babbling, was polite and gently reassuring. Looking back, what I really needed was for someone to grab me by the shoulders, tell me I was being insane and shake some sense into me. But it's hard for people to know how to respond when they are confronted by someone behaving so strangely.

At the wedding disco the next night I remember being on the dancefloor, a little pissed, jumping about to Dolly Parton's '9 to 5' and starting to feel just a tiny bit better, when I spied my cousin Joe on the other side of the room. We were close when we were little kids but I hadn't seen him much over the past decade. He was now a big-shot corporate lawyer, so I made a beeline straight for him; before he could offer to shake my hand or ask me how I was I had launched into a long, detailed monologue about the letter from HMRC. What made it worse for him was that the music was really loud, so he only heard every fourth or fifth word I was shouting at him: 'Dividends . . . self-assessment . . . prison food . . .' He looked back at my mad, bug-eyed face and tried to formulate a response. Luckily for him, my wife spotted what was going on and ushered me away politely. I was sent back to our bedroom alone to reflect on things. It didn't help.

There was more weird behaviour that went down on that beautiful, criminally wasted weekend in the Italian sunshine that I could tell you about, but you get the picture. I was mad. I had been triggered into an elongated panic attack by the arrival of a letter that turned out to be of little consequence whatsoever. I had a serious problem. But it wasn't with my tax affairs – it was with my brain.

* * *

I had always been an obsessive worrier. But I had learned how to hide it because shitting yourself about life's daily challenges was not really compatible with the hard-drinking, loud-talking superlad image I had been cultivating since I was about four.

My brain was busy all the time – I decided during the early stages of adulthood that the only way of avoiding any problems in life was to be on the lookout for them 100 per cent of the time. That way, you could spot them before they happened and take measures to fend them off. In other words, if you low-key shit yourself about stuff constantly then bad things will probably never happen. What a demented design for life that is.

Shrinks call it catastrophising.

It is tied into other forms of panic attack, like those times I would wake up in the night convinced that the small throb in my balls meant certain cancer or the stubborn zit on my back was an inoperable tumour.

If I wasn't worrying about something it meant I wasn't taking life seriously. It meant I was being complacent about the future and that something awful would inevitably happen to me because I had taken my eye off the ball.

I'm not entirely sure why my brain worked this way for so many years. But it doesn't any more. That's because I gave up drink and drugs. Ironically, these were the substances that I thought could combat constant worry. And while they sometimes chilled me out in the short term, they always made the worry come back twice as bad.

But more importantly, it was the lessons that sobriety taught me that helped. In therapy or AA or wherever else you seek help, you will learn three simple lessons that redefine your worldview:

127

1. Identify the stuff in life that you cannot control.
2. Let go of worrying about that stuff.
3. Take one day at a time.

This is why, in many ways, I consider my descent into problem drinking in my late thirties as a bit of a result.

Had I not reached the desperate point at which I had to seek help from people who knew about this stuff and had been through it themselves, I would never have learned those three lessons. I would have continued trying to wing my way through life. I would have continued to waste time worrying about what the future might bring, flying from one set of anxieties to the next, trying to navigate my way through with the numbing accompaniment of Kronenbourg and charlie.

Turns out, the big lessons of life had been staring me in the face all along. They were there hidden in the lexicon of football – where managers challenging for league titles repeatedly say that they are 'focusing on their own form . . . and taking each game as it comes'.

That is all you can do. The manager of Manchester United cannot control the form of Liverpool or Man City. He will gain nothing from staying awake all night fretting about the abilities of Liverpool's front three. It would be pointless. All he can do is coach his own players the best he can. And there is no point worrying about what might happen in three, four or six games' time. He can only prepare his players for the next fixture. Everything else is wasted mental energy.

If I had a time machine to go back to that weekend in Tuscany in August 2010, I might tell myself that I should just read that letter from HMRC properly and not speculate about what it might mean. I might tell myself that the conduct of my accountant was out of my hands and that all I needed to do was make sure my own affairs were in order. I might even grab myself by the shoulders and say: *You are fucking barmy, mate! You are doing everyone's head in! Pack it in and stop being so self-absorbed!* But, probably, I would just tell myself not to bother opening the letter in the first place. To just go to Italy and have a good time and worry about it when you get back. What difference do a couple of days make to anything anyway?

I can't go back and fix past mistakes.

But I can use the lessons of sobriety to help me through current challenges. I managed to get through the COVID pandemic without spiralling into a state of anxiety. In the past it certainly would have done. I am in a more privileged position than most. But I have managed to keep my head straight, my mood calm and my smile intact by falling back on these lessons: don't worry about future problems that will probably never arise; have faith in your ability to deal with shit if it ever does happen; and just try to focus on today. Look at the smaller picture, not the bigger one. The wider your perspective, the bigger scope there is to worry.

I hope you never have to experience problems with drink or drugs. But I do think everyone can learn valuable lessons from the process of recovery. Fuck tomorrow, it only really exists to mess with our minds.

12

The Day I Arranged to
Fight a Stranger

It was April 2015, just a few weeks before the general election, when I arranged to meet a complete stranger outside a tube station for a bare-knuckle fist fight.

It's the sort of thing you read about in football hooligan memoirs. But we were not hooligans. We were simply two middle-aged dads who disagreed over the nuances of government spending policy. It started as a reasonably intelligent debate, with both parties exchanging actual data on spending growth in relation to inflation and other dull crap. But eventually we both realised that no amount of facts and figures was going to resolve our disagreement so we decided to have a fight instead.

Things escalated quickly.

Before long we were exchanging direct messages. The arrangements went into quite advanced detail with the pair of us coordinating our schedules in order to meet and engage in physical combat.

This was no bluff on my part. In that moment, I was completely certain of my intentions to meet this bloke outside a central London tube station and fight him on the pavement. I went as far as explaining, in some detail, precisely what I would do to him once we had entered the arena of combat. Something about kicking him in the bollocks then knocking him out. With a single punch. This was designed to scare him but, in retrospect, was an unnecessary flourish that only made me more vulnerable. I mean, I doubt Bobby Fischer sent Boris Spassky written notice of his offensive strategy the day before a big chess match.

But it didn't matter because – as you'll have probably guessed – the fight never took place. We scheduled it for twenty-four hours hence – both claiming that the other party would be too much of a 'shitbag' to turn up. Ironically, neither of us did. At least I didn't and I'm assuming he didn't either or he would have been straight back on Twitter to call me out for my cowardice. As it was, we never exchanged messages again.

I guess I just somehow managed to calm down.

A good job too because I suppose I might have got beaten up (it hadn't occurred to me at the time that this bloke might be a bit handy). Mind you, the price I paid was mental rather than physical. I had lost twenty-four hours of my life consumed by rage, frustration and that strange social media anxiety you get where you can't stop checking your phone to see if some dickhead you've never met has messaged you back yet.

Those were twenty-four hours that I could have spent doing all sorts of more enjoyable things like playing with my kids, watching telly with my wife, walking in the park, reading a book, calling my mum, having a nice cup of tea, stroking my cat, doing the hoovering or eating some crisps.

* * *

How had I reached the point where I was planning to fight a stranger in a public place?

My drinking had filled me with so many bad thoughts and feelings that I needed constant distraction. Social media was an easy outlet for my anger and frustration.

I have always been quite politically minded and, as a general election loomed, I had become more and more absorbed in the daily debate. I felt angry about certain things I read in the news, frustrated that I couldn't change them and resentful towards the people who didn't seem to share my point of view. I was a walking embodiment of futile emotion.

On top of all that, I had slipped on an escalator at Camden Town tube station on my way home one night (following a solo sake binge in a branch of YO! Sushi during my lunchbreak) and broken my wrist pretty badly. After they operated, the doctors had given me some of those super-strong, prescription painkillers. I was popping them like they were Minstrels every day, washing them down with copious amounts of booze and substantial cocaine chasers. I should have just quit a couple of my jobs and simplified my life a little bit. I would have had more time on my hands, been less stressed and could have coped with the reduced income because I would have been giving less dough to the dealer and the publicans.

Those were the things I could have taken control over (I just didn't see it clearly enough at the time). What I had no control over was the political landscape, the management of the economy or the opinions of other, equally angry and frustrated people I met on Twitter.

I had enough to cope with in my own life and should have just focused on that stuff. Allowing myself to become so preoccupied and emotional about the things I saw on the news or read in the papers, then raging about it at anonymous people online, was about as helpful as going outside and shouting complaints at the moon for its inconvenient scheduling of the tides.

I've got mates who are regularly triggered by the news; stories about Brexit, COVID, Trump or whatever make them depressed or angry or both. I know that feeling. That's why I quit the news some time ago. I had to stop worrying about things I can't control. I have a general idea of what's going on in the world. But opinions and debate (which is what constitutes more than half of news coverage these days anyway) are not for me. That way madness lies. I used to host a national drivetime radio phone-in for three hours a day. It was exhausting and futile but just two years of doing that job was enough to put me off news chat for ever. In that sense, I'm grateful.

Most news nowadays is at least 40 per cent entertainment and/or clickbait. No one wants headlines that reflect the dreary ambiguity of most news stories. They don't want uncertain or vanilla headlines about Brexit or COVID. They want either doomsday predictions or Churchillian superlatives. Most of all, news outlets and their audiences want big, outrageous opinions and wild-eyed, bloodthirsty debates.

And you, as someone who probably has enough on your plate already, are collateral damage caught in the crossfire of all this bollocks. You are the bloke worrying about getting home to put the kids to bed while actively seeking out the viewpoints of people online who disagree with you about immigration or the NHS or fisheries. It is not your fault. You have been drip-fed fear and fury, conflict and poison, invective and hyperbole by a mixture of desperate media outlets who are running out of ways to make money and the millions of mad individuals on social media who will say and do anything to make themselves feel seen in a world where most of us are just helpless spectators.

Maybe you should make peace with being a helpless spectator.

You cannot control the news. Certainly not by worrying about it non-stop or entering useless debates with people whose minds you will never change.

You can only really control the way in which you live your own life. Try your best to live it in line with the values that you think are important. And if you want to run for office or start a campaign or write an era-defining treatise on the future of liberal democracy then by all means give it a crack. But look after your own feelings and mental health first. Delete Twitter, stop reading the news and take a break from forming opinions about everything that has ever happened. At least until you've got yourself sorted out. I got so embroiled in that world that I was actually trying to fight strangers over a difference of opinion. There is a self-absorption in that sort of behaviour that is really quite pathetic and unappealing in retrospect. The idea that my point of view is so important that it's worth punching someone over. Sometimes, the easiest way to get through a bad day is to look back on how much worse things used to be and remind yourself of the progress you have made.

13

The Numerous Things
I Have Failed At

I have been a freelancer for the best part of my twenty-five-year career. Throughout that time, I've been lucky enough to have been offered a diverse range of professional opportunities – most of which I have accepted instantly in the spirit of *Fuck it, I'll give it a go*. Some of them I have enjoyed, some of them not so much – but I have always come away having learned something useful. There is something to be said for having a go at everything. But there are also drawbacks – the more stuff you try, the more exposed you are to failure. I have failed at stuff many times.

When I was sixteen I walked into the coolest clothes shop in my local high street and asked for a Saturday job, which they gave me on the spot. I went round bragging to all my mates about how I had begun a career in the fashion industry. But on my first day in the shop, I made a grand total of zero sales. Then, while cleaning up at the end of the day, I managed to bust open the vacuum cleaner and release a large cloud of black dust all over the expensive clobber. I was immediately relieved of my duties.

As I've mentioned, I was a magazine-obsessed kid and when I left uni I was on a mission to get a job working for one. I was lucky to get a foot in the door at *Men's Health* – not quite the *Face*, admittedly, but a magazine all the same and, at the time, a successful one too. I learned loads from all the brilliant people on the editorial team. Turned out working on a mag was just as exciting as I had hoped. I was hooked on the business.

By the time I was in my mid-twenties I was deputy editor of a glossy monthly called *Later*. I got to interview superstars and my personal heroes from the worlds of music, sport and the movies. I had a brilliant boss and the rest of the team became good mates. We had so much fun. It was incredible. But when a mad Irish millionaire rocked up in London with dreams of launching a brand-new magazine and offered me the editor's job, I said yes without a moment's hesitation. That was how I was when I was younger: if the offer was there and the money was right, I would jump at it without thinking twice.

But this madman's idea for a new magazine was not a good one. For a start, it wasn't really a magazine at all. It was a CD-ROM that would be sold on the newsstand in WHSmith mounted on a magazine-shaped cardboard facade. He claimed it was a magazine that 'came to life' but, in fact, it turned out to be dead on arrival. The CD-ROM, once you loaded it on to your PC, gave access to various live-action interviews, games and videos. What a fucking stupid idea. I mean, in my defence, it was the year 2000. But to be honest, even back then CD-ROMs were a dated technology. The 'mag' lasted two issues before the company collapsed and I was left jobless and skint.

I had thought too much about being an editor on a big salary and not enough about what I wanted to do with my life. In the meantime, I had at least managed to hire three of my best mates as staff (yeah, they were well grateful when the whole thing went immediately tits up) and wasted loads of the Irish millionaire's money on plush West End offices and a massive Shoreditch launch party for which I hired a breakdance crew from Birmingham and flew in a Swedish funk band. I also commissioned a six-foot by six-foot ice sculpture of the brand logo that cost a grand and turned into a puddle before the party was over.

So, I can't say I was completely blameless in the premature collapse of the CD-ROM venture. But even if I had been completely studious in my approach to the job it was always destined to fail. Nobody wanted or needed a CD-ROM magazine. Not then, not now, not ever. Nevertheless, as I was sitting alone in my flat in the lonely weeks and months that followed the company's implosion, I found myself confronting feelings of professional failure for the first time since I'd got sacked from that clothes shop.

When shit goes bad in your life it can be helpful to examine your own role in the situation. It helps you grow, improves the quality of your future decisions and, above all, stops you becoming the sort of prick who blames everyone other than himself. Honest self-reflection is important.

But there is a big difference between self-reflection and self-flagellation. Branding yourself a failure is an easy but stupid thing to do. Failure is a big word. It sounds definitive and final. Like you've had a fair crack at something and been found, categorically and empirically, to be absolutely shit at it.

When you start thinking of yourself as a failure you go to a really dark place. You stop thinking of your problems as temporary challenges or natural bumps in the road and start seeing them as evidence of fundamental flaws in your character. Once those thoughts set in, you can expose yourself to really destructive feelings of self-doubt. In my experience those feelings mutate into depression quite easily. You can freeze completely, unable to muster the confidence or belief to get back out there and try to pursue even the smallest ambition ever again. In that state of mind you can make very bad decisions.

Just after my wife and I had our first child, I landed a job as the presenter of a TV documentary series about foreign criminal gangs operating in the UK. It was well paid and exciting. I had to interview south London Yardies, Turkish ex-heroin barons and undercover cops. On one particularly memorable day's filming I got to accompany the Berkshire police force on a drug raid of a skunk farm in Reading. Yes, friends, I was living the dream.

But after a few weeks' filming it became clear I wasn't cut out for the role. I was supposed to be a hard-nosed reporter, taking foreign criminals to task over the way they had 'infected' British society with their vile activities. Truthfully, though, I was often wide-eyed and excited by my encounters with gangsters. And, sometimes, I was even sympathetic to them. When the police nicked the young Chinese lad who had been overseeing the skunk farm in Reading he started to cry. The director told me to go and question him on his criminal activities but I ended up hugging him and telling him it would all be OK. The next day, my agent called and told me I was being replaced as the presenter. The production company thought I didn't have the right journalistic approach.

On reflection, they were right to sack me.

But at the time all I could do was sink into a swamp of misery. I was stung by the rejection and branded myself a failure. Not just a professional failure but worse – a failure as a father. The job had been easy in most respects. Filming interviews with cops and robbers is fun and thrilling, and the producers usually got me a taxi to and from the location. And yet I had fucked it up. I thought about all the other dads out there with proper jobs that required serious toil and long hours of boredom who just kept their heads down and got the work done because they had to provide for their families. I compared myself to those sorts of blokes and felt like a piece of shit. I let that thought really take hold and drag me down for a long period of time, during which I was unable to get back up, brush myself down and look forward to the next opportunity. My confidence fell out of my arse, I became utterly despondent and started looking for bar work.

By this stage in my life I had already been a journalist for over ten years and had some success behind me. I was miles off the point at which I should have been contemplating a complete career change. I had just hit a temporary setback. But the voice in my head whispering 'failure' was relentless and kept getting louder. Luckily, I had a wife who helped slowly to rebuild my paper-thin self-esteem and convince me it wasn't time just yet to start knocking out pints of Guinness down the Red Lion (not that there's anything wrong with that line of work – it just wasn't part of my career trajectory at the time).

I always tended to be a bit fragile.

As with the CD-ROM debacle, I had the capacity to overreact and beat myself up when I let good opportunities turn bad. But becoming a dad really exaggerated that tendency. TV and films tell us that good dads are responsible, hardworking and selfless. They are solid and consistent. They put their family before themselves in everything they do. So, when we don't conform to that narrow definition of successful fathering, we can be quick to start hating ourselves.

Then there is the slightly old-fashioned and sexist notion that fathers are supposed to 'provide' for their families. Despite my liberal, feminist posturing, I was as in thrall to this idea as the next idiot. I thought I had to not just provide food and shelter for my child, I had to give her a special childhood – or at least one more special than my own.

I was fixated on giving my daughter (and the son who came along a few years later) so much more than I had: endless holidays, takeaways, trips to Hamleys and loads and loads of bikes and *Star Wars* figures.

I set the bar unrealistically high and whenever I (inevitably) fell short I would demolish myself mentally and emotionally. I could no longer lose a bit of freelance work and just crack on. For the first few years of fatherhood even the expiry of a not particularly lucrative contract would sometimes send me spinning into long, tedious and exhausting periods of self-loathing and existential despair.

Fifteen years into fatherhood, I think I've got over all that now – more or less.

I will still judge myself harshly from time to time. If I fuck something up I will still occasionally catch myself mouthing the word 'wanker' at my own reflection in the bathroom mirror. But I am now able to shut those kinds of negative thoughts down quicker. I spot them early, know exactly where they might lead and make a very conscious decision to close them down before they take hold.

Sometimes I avoid negative thoughts by trying to distract my brain with other stuff – like happy memories or positive affirmations or football management games on the PlayStation.

Much more importantly than that, I judge myself on simpler terms these days. I try to focus on one clear version of myself and try to be the best at being that. Basically, I want to be a decent husband and father who is reliable and loving – and content. Being content in myself is important to being a decent father and husband. Those dads who keep their heads down and mouths shut and get on with their daily toil without any time for themselves usually end up being grumpy and miserable. Or having premature heart attacks. I look after my own happiness in simple ways these days: tea; cats; football; music. And if none of that works I can always smash the emergency glass and call upon the old failsafe: a wank and a Snickers.

When I was younger, I was often trying to be a million different people all at once. And all my different personas would end up getting in the way of each other. That meant I was often miserable. Nowadays, I know who I am. I don't set my standards that high; I don't need to be wildly rich or consistently ecstatic. I don't think I need to lavish my kids with treats and bikes and holidays to make me a good dad (in fact, I realise the reverse is probably true). When stuff to do with work sometimes goes iffy or I'm skint at the end of the month, I still feel a bit worried or gutted. But I don't start thinking of myself as a failure. I've got those daft thoughts on lockdown. I just think I'm a normal bloke having all the same ups and downs as everyone else. I realise that bad moments always pass and rarely, if ever, get remotely close to the mad catastrophes you conjure in your mind when you lie awake at night.

You could say I have successfully lowered my expectations of myself. Really, I have just come to recognise that the expectations should have been lower all along.

14

Drunk Dad

I didn't want to be a drunk dad. I didn't want to be a burnout husband who spent more time in the pub than at home. But by my late thirties that was what I was becoming.

My wife had watched on as my fun weekend drinking had morphed gradually into depressing, all-the-time drinking. She felt helpless. The kids weren't quite registering the problem yet but it was only a matter of time before it dawned on them that Dad was a hopeless pisshead. This is the part where I tell you that I got sober for them. That the deep love I felt for my wife and kids gave me the strength I needed to turn my life around. But that's not strictly true. More than anything, I got sober for myself. If I'd only done it for them I would have resented them for it and eventually relapsed anyway. I had to really, really want to give up drink for the sake of my own life.

I had known for over a year that I had pretty much lost control of my bad habits. I was not in denial about them. I was doing coke at work and getting pissed before lunch. I was sneaking around in ever-more elaborate ways to get wasted in secret amidst my everyday obligations. Pretending to have a cold or hay fever to explain the constant drip from my nose. Making up reasons to go to the shop so I could swing by the pub and neck a couple of double whiskies at high speed. Feigning stomach upsets in order to explain my frequent trips to the toilet. Sneaking out at night to hide my empties in litter bins two streets away. I could see quite clearly how depressing, weird and wrong all of this was. But by this stage my habits were teetering on the edge of pure addiction: no matter how much I wanted to stop, no matter how sad it all made me feel, I just kept on doing it day after day. If I stopped, the misery and panic and exhaustion would overwhelm me. I was scared of sobriety and the return of my depression.

My wife was not aware of the full extent of my problem because I was so secretive but she knew enough to have asked me to stop on numerous occasions as I entered the final year of my thirties. Every time she confronted me about my drinking – sometimes with tears in her eyes – I would tell her with the utmost seriousness that I was quitting for good. But even as I said it, I knew I was lying. The bad habits were just too important to me. They were a crutch that I didn't feel I could live without but I didn't expect her to understand that. So I thought it was better for everyone if I just bullshitted her and then continued to get wasted every day in secret. I would just have to work harder to hide my habits.

There were times when I convinced myself that using drugs and drink to get through the day actually made me a better family man. It regulated my mood and made me better able to cope with the mental exhaustion that might otherwise have engulfed me. Plus the drugs in particular gave me the physical energy to do all the shit I had to do.

And at that stage of my life, I had so much shit to do. When I turned thirty-nine, we had just bought a new house. But there was a six-month period where it was being renovated and effectively we had to sofa surf from one hospitable relative to the next. It was fun and novel for the first couple of weeks but then it just became stressful and tiring. At this time I was freaking out about money and work even more than usual. The new house, the renovations, the two kids – the costs were mounting up, I had got myself into all sorts of debt and I woke every morning with texts from the bank warning me about my overdraft. I was frantic and miserable.

I thought I could simply earn my way out of it all by taking on as much work as possible. I was lucky to have the opportunities to do so. I was finishing my third book, which was already long overdue with the publishers. I had taken on a fairly big executive position at a TV company. This was something I'd never done before and I didn't have a huge amount of passion for it. But I'd taken on the role because I needed some professional and financial security. It involved being back in a highly corporate environment to which I already knew, from my past experience in magazines, I wasn't suited. Rules and processes are not something I deal with very well. Nor are bosses. A more professional person than me would have sucked it up, found a way of fitting in and just got the job done anyway. But I was not particularly professional. So I became angry and petulant and then sought solace in drugs and booze, which I would consume every day to numb my feelings of frustration and alienation.

During half-term I invited my daughter, then aged seven, to join me at the office one day. I was the boss of a department and assumed it would be fine to have her there quietly drawing at my desk for the day. But when I arrived at the building with her by my side, an unannounced guest in this high-security compound that passed for a media outfit, all hell broke loose. Someone from HR confronted me angrily in front of my daughter, reading out a list of the rules and protocols I had broken by bringing her in without consent. My daughter, distraught at the idea that she had got me into trouble, burst into tears. The HR person looked at her blankly, then told us both to leave the building.

So we did. I should never have gone back after that but when my boss heard about the incident she apologised to me and smoothed things over. I went back the next day but was unhappier and more resentful than ever. I hated the culture there. None of which was an excuse for my drinking or drug abusing, of course. I mean, there were a million more positive responses to a shit job than becoming an addict. But I was not thinking straight. I had put myself under too much financial pressure and I allowed myself to believe that I was trapped in that situation. I did have a way out. But I was never going to be able to find it while I was off my face.

At the same time as working at the TV company, I was freelancing as a presenter for a couple of national radio stations. I didn't have my own regular show at the time – I was the guy who covered the other hosts when they were sick or on holiday. Sometimes this sort of work would come in at short notice. But it was quite well paid and lots of fun so I felt I couldn't afford to turn it down. As a result, my average day in 2014 looked like this:

6 a.m. Get up, have breakfast with the kids.

8 a.m. Shower, get dressed and ride my moped six miles across London to my job at the TV company.

9 a.m.–11 a.m. Attend a series of pointless meetings with other

telly bosses and become embroiled in a passive-aggressive cold war with my colleagues.

11 a.m. Back on the moped to speed over to the radio studios on the other side of London (claiming to my TV colleagues that I was just 'popping out for a quick meeting').

1 p.m.–4 p.m. Present national radio show.

4 p.m. Ride back to the TV company in order to collect my bag and show my face at the end of the day. Luckily, no one there ever listened to the radio so they were completely unaware that I'd been moonlighting.

8 p.m. Arrive back at home, have dinner with the family before retreating to my office to work on my long-overdue book.

8 p.m.–3 a.m. Write frantically through the night while my family slept. Fuel myself through the long night with Jack Daniel's. Pop a Valium to nab three hours sleep before starting all over again the next morning.

It was an unsustainable way of living, clearly. It was also unnecessary. I had other options (something that so many other people don't). For a start, I could have just cut back on my overheads rather than try to increase my earnings to keep up. The booze, drugs and long lunches were probably accounting for the proceeds from all the extracurricular work I was doing anyway. But my mind was spinning: a mixture of fear, frustration and self-loathing. I didn't want to stop and get off the ludicrous rollercoaster I had created for myself. I just kept ploughing on.

Maybe if someone had intervened and told me I was overdoing it I might have listened. But my wife was cautious of telling me to slow down: whenever she tried, I would rant and rave, accusing her of not understanding the seriousness of our situation and the pressure I was under. All she wanted was for me to put myself first; she wanted us to find a way of organising our lives that didn't require me to behave like a madman all the time. I told her she was naive.

As for the other people who might have intervened – friends, family, colleagues – they just wouldn't have known about the depths of my problem. I was very good at putting on a positive, capable and accomplished front to everyone. As a freelancer, it was necessary: I needed each of my employers to think that they were my only priority. I couldn't show them how thinly I was stretching myself. I had too much pride to ever allow my family to think my drinking was out of control. I had relatives who had serious drinking problems, which everyone had been worried about for years. I didn't want to be a black sheep like them. I posed as the more measured and composed part of the family. Adopting that pose became increasingly taxing as my lifestyle became ever more destructive. There were Sunday lunches at my mum's where I would turn down a glass of wine, then leave the table, sneak into the living room and nab furtive gulps of Scotch from the bottle she kept in the cupboard. I always had a packet of Extra Strong Mints on me to disguise the ever-present whiff of alcohol on my breath.

Sometimes I would stay out after work, drinking with colleagues. Other times I would travel back to our little suburb alone and just set up camp in a quiet pub close to home. There I would spend a whole evening drinking alone, arriving home after my wife and kids had gone to bed. I had lost the thread. I wasn't enjoying any of this. I was sad all of the time. But I thought that I would be even sadder if I stopped.

I had been on anti-depressants for a few years already. I was also starting to develop something of a taste for max-strength painkillers. They helped with the incessant hangovers but they also started to become a general comfort that I made part of my daily toxin regime.

Probably the most painful memory of that time is when we went on holiday with a couple of other families. As far as my wife was concerned, I'd stopped drinking about a month beforehand. In reality, I had continued to booze heavily while doing a good job of hiding it from her. I had worked up an alcohol tolerance that allowed me to imbibe huge quantities of the stuff without showing any outward signs of inebriation.

But on the first night of the holiday, I decided to make use of the resort's all-inclusive offering. The other dads were hitting the cocktails hard and I figured it was fine to join in on the basis it was a 'special occasion'. Anna's face dropped the moment she saw me clutching a pina colada.

'What's the matter with you?' I asked, like a belligerent prick.

'Is that it then?' she asked. 'You're just drinking again?'

'I'm not drinking again. I am having one drink because I am on holiday and relaxing with my mates. Don't make such a big deal out of it.'

We both knew what I was saying was complete bollocks. I was daring her to make a scene in front of our pals and she understandably dropped the issue. But the next morning, when I woke up hung over in the room we were sharing with the kids, she was still angry. She didn't want to argue in front of the kids so she insisted nothing was the matter when I continually asked why she was acting so grumpy. I was feeling guilty and ashamed but those feelings suddenly burst out of me in the form of anger. I told her she was ruining the holiday. I told her she was uptight and boring. I said it was her who had the problem, not me. That I was a normal bloke who wanted to unwind – and she was a neurotic who wanted to control me.

As I write this down all these years later, I feel so ashamed. But I've spoken to enough recovering addicts since then to know that this state of rage and denial is so common in pissheads.

This was a woman who had loved me unconditionally for the past twenty years. She had changed my whole life by giving me the confidence and self-belief that I had lacked as a kid. She had done it by loving me. I had let her down badly. I was making her unhappy and scared. And when she tried to help me, I turned everything back on her. I wanted to make her feel guilty, as if she were the problem. Did I actually believe that in my addled mind? No. I think I was being very calculating and manipulative. My goal was to keep doing exactly what I wanted. I just wanted to carry on drinking all the time. Anna was a threat to that and I would say or do almost anything to get her out of my way. The love of my life. My best friend. The mother of my children. I still loved her but booze had me by the short and curlies and was telling me that all obstacles to our illicit affair had to be destroyed, or at least cowed into submission.

It was the one time my daughter was really exposed to how my drinking was starting to escalate into something scary. As I spiralled into a state of self-righteous fury, shouting all this horseshit at Anna in our little room, Coco started to cry and asked me to stop. But I didn't stop. I said something like: 'Sorry, Coco, but Mum thinks I'm crazy and doesn't like me any more.' My son, Len, was three years old and seemed completely distracted by *Peppa Pig* on the iPad. Perhaps he subconsciously absorbed the shouting and nastiness. I asked Coco recently if she remembered the incident and she said she didn't. But I know it shook her up at the time because I remember the tears streaming down her face and the pleading way in which she kept repeating the word 'Stop'. In the end, they left the room.

I calmed down and by the end of that day the whole thing was brushed under the carpet. We managed to have a nice holiday, at least on the surface. Deep down I knew my behaviour had been horrendous and unacceptable but I shielded myself from the guilt by channelling it into self-pity and indignance. Again, I have since learned this is a very common form of defence and denial among addicts.

I'm going through old boxes of my newspaper cuttings one afternoon, preparing to move into a new office. It's early spring 2022, and I have been sober for seven years. Life feels good. But the old articles from across the years relay a curious sort of biography. Although it is all self-penned, much of it was written at the behest of a publication or editor that had a certain agenda or angle they needed me to accommodate.

On the cover of a crumpled copy of the *Telegraph*'s 'Weekend' supplement, dated July 2013, there's a large colour image of me baking cakes with my two children, who were then aged six and eighteen months respectively. We are all laughing, seemingly enraptured in the bosom of wholesome familial love. There are eggs and flour on the table, both Waitrose own brand.

The image is partly authentic: they were my kids, it was my home and, yes, I did occasionally bake stuff with them. But the inauthentic parts had been contrived to satisfy the *Telegraph*'s fantasy about idyllic, middle-class family life. For a start, I was wearing my best shirt, which was freshly ironed. The kids were also in their best clothes. We were never, ever this smart or organised in any part of our lives, let alone a baking session. The Waitrose produce had been brought along by the photographer as props (we never shopped at Waitrose). And the flour on my face had been smudged there carefully for effect by a make-up artist. When I posted the image on Facebook one of my best mates commented underneath: 'Is that charlie all over your face?' At around that time in my life, it was just as likely to have been.

The headline reads DADZILLA: THE RISE OF THE SUPER DADS. The article is basically about what a modern, dynamic, loving and super-hands-on dad I was at the time. The tone is purposefully boastful. I claim at one point to be the 'best dad in the world'. It's fucking mad.

I stare at this picture for about five minutes, trying to get inside the head of that version of myself from nine years ago. Did I really think I was the best dad in the world? Was I really as loving, caring, jolly and capable as the article and accompanying image seemed to suggest? Of course not. Nobody is that dad in real life. Being a dad is fucking hard. For the first few years it can feel overwhelming. Yes, I spent a lot of time at home with the kids in those days because I was freelance and my wife worked full-time. I probably did more cooking, school-gate shifts and playground visits than most other dads I knew. And, some of the time, I really enjoyed it.

But a lot of the time I just felt lonely, exhausted, miserable and bored shitless. In the piece, I semi-admit to having had these feelings in my early days of fatherhood. But I claim that I overcame them by approaching my role in a super-masculine, competitive way. Not once did I mention that I was increasingly coping with the stress by getting solo pissed after my family went to bed at night or staying up doing loads of coke.

Rather than trying to make other dads feel inadequate by comparison I should have been telling the truth about the struggles of fatherhood. Dads don't talk to each other about that enough. Mums (who generally have it a lot tougher than us in every way) seem to be better at sharing the struggles of parenthood with each other. They are honest about how tough it is. And they seem less scared that, by admitting to this, they will somehow be perceived as less loving or competent.

Most young dads I know rush full steam into fatherhood and, all too often, hit a brick wall when they realise how unrelenting the pressures are. You lose almost all time to yourself for a couple of years and miss out on a ton of sleep, which is a sure-fire way to send you batty. This often manifests itself as self-pity, frustration, exhaustion and anger. Which, in turn, can lead some blokes (like me) into heavy drinking and/ or drugs as a means of blowing off steam.

Fatherhood is the best thing that ever happened to me. But it also presented me with some of the toughest challenges of my life. If I had been more honest about that – and other dads had been more honest with me about their own experiences – I would have had fewer feelings of guilt or inadequacy. I might have been less likely to fall into addiction.

If you're a younger dad or a would-be father reading this, I hope I'm not putting you off. All I would say is that fatherhood is hard – if you're doing it right. A lot of dads just simply fuck off when the going gets tough. If you stick around and put a shift in then you are a hero. But when it knackers you (which it will) try to look after yourself, be honest with yourself, share your struggles with other parents who may be going through the same thing and don't seek solace in booze or other bad stuff. Acknowledge that what you're going through is tough and that you deserve to feel tired but don't let that mutate into self-pity. That will only make you angry with the world and turn you into a bit of a dickhead. It did with me. I was working hard to be a good dad but was kind of pissed off that nobody had given me a medal. The more I drank, the angrier and more self-pitying I became. It's a vicious circle.

PART 2
SOBER

15

The Day I Stopped Drinking

On 25 June 2015 I drove up to the Priory rehab centre in London and turned myself in.

I was forty years old and realised enough was enough. I had been on the piss every day for months. I was sometimes drinking before midday. (By 'sometimes' I mean 'often'. And by 'midday' I mean 'ten in the morning'.)

Anna had gone from tolerance to annoyance to anger to deep concern over the course of the past year. I had gone from delusion to defensiveness to rage to despair in the same period. Now I was just sick of myself and the endless cycle of sordid inebriation and lies I was trapped inside. Plus I was fat and skint and miserable, and for the first time had started to contemplate the possibility that I might drop dead at any moment, leaving my two kids fatherless.

By the time you realise you have to stop drinking, it's too late to do it alone.

The most important thing about 'coming out' as a full-blown pisshead is that you make yourself accountable. By finally admitting to everything and telling everyone you're stopping for good, you take away the secrecy. Everyone is watching you. People you love are rooting for you. There are fewer places to hide. Or to put it another way:

Once you've gone round loudly telling everyone you've stopped drinking then you're going to look like twice the dickhead if you fall off the wagon.

There had, of course, been numerous stops and starts. The odd dry fortnight here and there. But all that sort of sporadic abstinence does is falsely convince you that you have some control over the situation.

I didn't have control.

I would reward myself for managing to stay sober all week by getting absolutely shitfaced on Friday night. Madness.

At the Priory, they gave me a free assessment. I had booked the appointment online a few days earlier, in the dead of night, wide awake and frantic with anxiety and self-loathing, my wife sleeping beside me. Why did I choose the Priory? Because it was near where I lived. And also I had heard of it – it's the fancy showbiz rehab place that's always mentioned in the papers.

I met a therapist who asked me to describe my drinking and drug taking over the past couple of weeks. Obviously, my first instinct was to lie about that. But how mad would it be to go and seek help for drink and drugs then bullshit the person who was trying to help you? She made things much easier by explaining that she was a recovering addict herself. 'Whatever you've done, however bad you think your behaviour has been, I've probably done stuff twice as bad. So don't hold back,' she said. I liked her from the start. She is still my therapist today.

So I told her about every drink I'd had over the past two weeks and all the drugs and stupidity that had gone along with them. She nodded, non-judgementally, but told me that I clearly had a problem.

She gave me a no-fucking-about choice: I could either resolve to stop drinking completely, in which case she could help me. Or I could decide to try and moderate my drinking, in which case she couldn't. Because once you've become a problem drinker, the ability to moderate is just a barmy dream. One glass of wine with dinner on a Saturday night? Good luck with that, mate.

How do you know if you're a problem drinker? Where is the line between being a good-times drinker who likes a few pints and couple of cheeky lines a few times a week, and a problematic drinker on a runaway train towards total oblivion? Hard to say. But I increasingly believe that if you think you might have a problem then you definitely do have a problem.

Just don't wait for the so-called 'rock bottom' moment to arrive before you decide to do something about it. Because by then it might be too late to ever fix yourself. Plus, it might never come. There are plenty of people who have managed to avoid death, incarceration, extreme violence or the collapse of their career while maintaining a horrible booze problem that has nevertheless made them and those around them completely miserable. Functioning alcoholics are everywhere. I bet you can immediately think of at least three to whom you're pretty close.

You don't need to be a park-bench drinker to be an alcoholic. You just have to be someone who regularly decides they don't want to drink but then finds themselves doing it anyway. And then feels shit about it afterwards.

Meeting my therapist and hearing her talk about her experiences of addiction and recovery, and being able to share all the bad habits and terrible feelings that had started to define my life, made me understand that I had a problem that had to be nipped in the bud. I, like most other drinkers, had underestimated the extent of the problem for too long. She combined just the right amounts of understanding and brutality to shake me to my senses.

In the car on the way home I decided I was going to never drink again.

I haven't had a single drop of alcohol since.

I didn't become an inpatient at the Priory but started seeing her once a week to keep myself on track.

I don't want to make it sound easy. It isn't, and there were all sorts of other challenges to combat over the weeks and months that followed. I still face them today. Drink, drugs and all the other destructive habits we use are usually symptoms of a deeper pain that we've failed to deal with in more constructive ways.

Until recent years, we couldn't really admit to anyone that we felt that sort of pain because we feared it would make us sound weird or weak or whingey. So we had to bury it deep inside and, whenever it tried to rear its head and start causing trouble, silence it with drink, drugs or whatever.

I am aware that I promised not to offer too much advice in this book. All I am trying to do is share my own experiences in the hope that they might resonate with others. But here I am offering more advice – please feel free to completely ignore it and skip to the next story about me acting like a prick. In any case, here's what I advise anyone who is serious about quitting drink: make yourself accountable. Admit the full extent of your habits to someone. If not someone close to you then someone who has been there and done that. That's why Alcoholics Anonymous works for so many people. You won't get judged and there are people who have already fought the battles that you are fighting now.

Don't get all worried if they start talking about God at AA.

They don't mean God out of the Bible. They mean the invisible forces that make life so terrifyingly arbitrary. Getting your head around the inherent unpredictability of human existence – and just sort of learning to accept it without resorting to boshing four pints of Kronenbourg every lunchtime – is really at the heart of all this.

Sounds tough, right? But once you start thinking about this stuff, just a little bit every day, then I promise you life gets easier, happier and more peaceful. I sleep like a baby every night and have done consistently since 25 June 2015. In the immortal words of Joe Fagin, that's living all right.

16

Cocaine Is Just the Worst

The older I get, the more I realise that keeping things simple is the key to happiness. Don't overcomplicate life. Slowing down and being still is a super-cure for so many of our problems. Not full-time, obviously. None of us is Buddha. Bills need paying, the kitchen needs cleaning and the cat wants feeding. That said, an ability to embrace peace, react to things calmly and just take a breath once in a while is the best shot any of us have of avoiding complete meltdown. No, I'm not saying you have to start doing yoga. Just switching your phone off in the evening is a start. I am totally convinced of this. French philosopher Blaise Pascal once said, 'All of humanity's problems stem from man's inability to sit quietly in a room alone.' Bloody right. If we could all just tap the brakes a bit more we'd be better off for it.

The antithesis of this design-for-life is called cocaine.

Cocaine is a powder you snort (or smoke, or – if you're a seventies rock star – have blown up your bumhole through a McDonald's straw by a flunky) that immediately, magically, makes you the opposite of peaceful, calm and still.

When you take coke you become instantly anxious, noisy and intense. It is a poison: it corrupts everything inside your body, your mind and your soul. It makes you aggressively boring – babbling to anyone who will listen about your idea for the world's first electric cricket bat or how much you love Oasis's third album.

But you know all this, right? Because you, like me and everyone else, have done loads of cocaine. Seriously, every fucker in Britain over the age of twelve has been bang on the gear for years now. The days of cocaine being a designer drug for yuppies ended forty years ago. What about the builders, the taxi drivers, the football hooligans, the call-centre workers and the unemployed teenagers who are all bang at it? Let alone the royals, the politicians, the tired-out mums, the stressed-out dads, the teachers, the doctors, the butchers, the bakers, the candlestick makers and – of course – the chefs (chefs love coke). Britain is collectively hooked on beak.

Mate, even your grandparents have done cocaine.

But no one really likes doing coke, do they? We all know it makes you edgy and paranoid and twattish. It's not even as if the grim consequences are deferred to the next morning like booze and other drugs. Within hours of doing cocaine, you find yourself lying awake, sweaty and terrified in your bed, feeling more alone and worthless than you ever imagined possible. You know that's what it does to you and yet you still hand over sixty quid you can't afford for the pleasure. Cocaine defies every marketing orthodoxy known to humankind.

So why does everyone keep taking it?

Maybe it's because we're all so knackered all the time. Maybe you're exhausted from work or from raising kids or both. Or maybe you're woozy from all the beer you've drunk in the pub. I got to the stage where I couldn't contemplate having any more than two pints without making sure I had at least a gram either in my pocket or on its way in an Uber.

It's no coincidence that coke made its big breakthrough in Thatcher's decade when we were all brainwashed into thinking that personal productivity was the only measure of human value and that rampant ambition was a desirable lifestyle choice.

Cocaine can be a useful accompaniment to those sort of warped life goals. If you're the kind of person who wants to 'work hard, play hard' then cocaine helps sustain your unnatural and wholly unsustainable lifestyle choices. Cocaine is not even meant to be fun to take – like ecstasy or weed or even (I'm told) heroin. It's simply a means to an end. It will get you through a working day or a drunken evening without the need for a lie down.

In my late thirties I came to rely on coke like asthmatics rely on their inhalers. It was no longer a weekend treat: it was a daily necessity. I didn't even associate it with having fun any more. I associated it with getting stuff done. I was constantly trying to give up. But I got locked into a cycle of abstinence and relapse. Sometimes these cycles would take place in a mere matter of hours. I would buy some cocaine, do a couple of lines, feel immediately shit about myself and throw the rest away in a street bin. Then, about an hour or two later when the effects of the initial lines wore off and I started to feel jittery, I would call the dealer and buy some more. The frustration and self-loathing this mad behaviour stirred inside me made the numbing release of more cocaine even more appealing. It was a rough time.

The simplest way to describe how I went from an absolutely fucking tragic cokehead in my late thirties to seven years sober is this: I just started allowing myself to have that lie down.

I realised pressing pause and lying down for a bit was not a cop out. It was, in fact, a magical and life-affirming cure all. If you want to get ahead, have a kip, mate. That's my advice.

No one likes hearing other people's drug stories so I will keep mine as brief as I can. I saw a lot of cocaine snorting when I was a kid but I can't say it ever became normalised. I found it terrifying no matter how many times I saw it done. I didn't see much of a difference between the grim spectacle of Zammo chasing the dragon in *Grange Hill* and someone hoovering a line of bugle off my mum's coffee table.

Then when I was in my mid-teens my best mate and I somehow embroiled ourselves in the stag do of a fella ten years our senior. He and all of his mates were MEN who did MANLY things on this stag – like having sex with women and taking cocaine. I was just a bewildered spectator. We ended up back at someone's flat partying and I fell asleep, pissed out of my head. When I woke up my best mate was striding rapidly around the living room clutching his nose and saying, 'OOOooooooowwwwww, fuck!' He told me he had tried cocaine and was in immense pain. Which wasn't much of an advertisement for it, really. But you know how it is when you're a teenager: my mate had tried it so now I had to.

When I got to university a couple of years later it was something I started doing most weekends when the loan stretched to it. In my twenties, I joined the glittering world of the London media where living at a fast pace and acting like a bit of a cunt seemed de rigueur – and cocaine helped you do both.

I would sometimes go a year or two without touching the stuff.

That's how it tricks you into thinking you have agency. It was in my mid to late thirties that things got out of hand. I stopped using it for 'fun' and started using it as a crutch to get me through an increasingly taxing and stressful life. That's not an excuse, by the way. Not everyone with those roles to perform resorts to narcotic support. Some people are able to balance their lives, attain perspective and just, you know, not do loads of coke all the time. But I didn't because I was stupid and had a distorted idea of what life was all about.

Throughout those final years of my cocaine use, I can honestly say I never once actually enjoyed the sensation it gave me. I was quite simply hooked: I had forgotten how to function without it. When I finally got clean for good, a lot of mates – most of whom were the people I used to do coke with and probably felt a bit uncomfortable with my abstinence – scoffed at the idea that I was an addict. They told me I just had a 'bad habit'. As if having a bad habit was perfectly OK. Habit, addiction, call it what you want – but shovelling gear up your hooter in the disabled bogs at 9 a.m. to prepare for a meeting is not the behaviour of someone who is delighted by his own life choices or confident about the way the future is going to unfold.

You might still be doing gear and thinking to yourself, *That all sounds fucking seedy and depressing whereas my drug use is fun and social and glamorous.* But cocaine is a powerful, deceptive and sadistic substance that will fool you into thinking you have control until – BAM! – you don't. Just like booze, it is a noose tightening slowly around your neck. By the time you can't breathe any more, it's too late to wrestle free. Fun times soon give way to paranoid solo binges, frantic late-night desperation calls to dealers who secretly pity you and that terrible, constant worry that the person you are talking to can see traces of white powder caked around your nostrils.

Urgh. Cocaine sucks.

But the weird thing is that, of my two addictions, coke is the one I fear most. I can recall the warm glow that booze would sometimes give me and yet I never really miss it. I never crave an alcoholic drink – the thought sickens me. Whereas I know that cocaine could work its way back into my life at any moment if I don't stay vigilant. Cocaine is something I have nothing but negative memories of. From that first line I ever did to the last, it brought me nothing but discomfort, fear and regret. And yet I know it's still there, lurking in the shadows of my mind, waiting to lure me back into its toxic embrace at the first chance it gets.

I am Dot Cotton and cocaine is my Nick.

This is why I take recovery seriously, even after all these years. Complacency can easily set in and my addictions are always waiting for another chance to get started. So I share with other people who have been through the same sort of experiences; I go to therapy to talk through the feelings that once led me down those dark paths; I keep myself fit and healthy; and, perhaps most importantly of all, I rest. Fuck 'the grind', fuck 'work hard, play hard' and fuck Thatcher. These are inhuman forces that, if you're not careful, can drive you into the arms of the dope man.

17

This Is What an Addict Looks Like

For about three years after I first gave up drinking, one of my relatives had this habit of offering me wine every single time I went round for dinner. I would politely decline and she would always act surprised and say: 'Really? Are you driving?'

'No,' I'd reply. 'I don't drink any more. Remember?'

'I barely drink myself these days,' she'd say and then proceed to tell me in prolonged detail about the ins and out of her modest weekly booze schedule.

This is a common response when you first tell people you don't drink. They seem to think you need to hear about their own habits. Sometimes they sound insistent, like they think you don't believe them when they tell you about how they only drink at weekends (massive yawn). Or they sound defensive, as if they think you might be judging them.

But, in my case, they needn't worry about either of those things. The truth is, I just sincerely don't give a shit about how or when other people drink. It's their business. And it's fucking boring.

Sometimes they ask: 'Why don't you drink?'

Sometimes, in the early days, I would just say something glib like: 'I just sleep better,' or 'It's not for ever – I just took a couple of weeks off and liked the way it felt so carried on.'

I wanted to be accountable and open about why I'd stopped. But sometimes I just couldn't be bothered going into it. Back then, it sometimes just felt awkward to tell the truth.

If you're in a social situation, people don't want to hear you explain your abstinence by saying, 'Unaddressed childhood trauma combined with a deep sense of inadequacy, mate. Got any elderflower cordial?'

Not only did they not want to hear about the deeper psycho-emotional issues that underpinned my addictions, I didn't want to think about them either. I began sober life by convincing myself that I'd just let things get out hand and that total abstinence was the only way out. Which was superficially true. But there were all sorts of other, deeper things that needed addressing in order to understand why I became a pisshead in the first place. Only by understanding them could I confront them and, hopefully, set myself free. It's not easy to do that – but it's easier than being enslaved by the need to drink or snort your feelings away every evening.

If you're thinking about giving up booze but reckon all that 'confronting your feelings' stuff sounds like a bit of a hassle, all I would say is that it's not nearly as much of a hassle as trying to sort out your Uber home from the pub after throwing up on your shoes.

You might think that you drink to relax but once you get sober and look back, drinking just seems like such a massive pain in the arse. Being pissed is confusing and uncomfortable, and being hung over is even worse. Every simple task becomes more difficult. You're almost always knackered. Also, you're always worried about how much of a cunt you might be making of yourself. At least these days I am fully aware of what a cunt I am making of myself.

People seemed so grateful when I played down my drinking.

The last thing they wanted was for me to say I had a drink problem. Because if I did, perhaps they did. And if they did then maybe they would have to do something about it.

People like to believe that alcoholics are only the tramps on park benches drinking meths. They want to think of drug addicts like Nick Cotton clucking for skag in *EastEnders*. They need to believe that addicts are completely alien. But addicts do come in all shapes and sizes. We are not all shitting the bed every night or getting arrested for trying to fuck a bin bag on Clapham Common. We are functioning. We are living seemingly normal, often successful lives – but secretly anaesthetising ourselves from the turmoil inside our heads with habitual drinking and drug taking. Until we admit we have a problem, ask for help and start living a happier life in which we are unlikely to ever shit the bed or put our cocks inside a refuse sack.

Nowadays, I know who I am.

I know my flaws. I embrace my vulnerabilities. I know I can be a bit of a dickhead. But I am comfortable in my own skin. I am what an addict looks like: six-foot-two, bald and fucking gorgeous, mate.

After three years of being offered wine by this relative – who seemed to delight in 'forgetting' that I was teetotal – I'd had enough. One day she offered me a drink over lunch and I went through the usual routine of reminding her that I didn't drink but this time, when she said: 'Remind me why you stopped?' I replied, dead casual like, 'Because I was a massive alcoholic and cokehead.'

That shut her up.

18

Fear Made Me Drunk.
Love Got Me Sober

Until 25 June 2015, I'd been sleepwalking through life.

It might have looked as if I was doing all right. I had a career and a family. I seemed to be successful and happy. And I really was happy a lot of the time. I didn't turn into a pisshead because I was constantly miserable. I turned into a pisshead because I was scared. I was scared of what people thought about me and scared of what might happen if all the good stuff in my life suddenly disappeared. I gave off the impression of being super-confident in myself. But deep down inside I was pretty convinced that the happy life I had built could collapse at any moment. And when it did I would not know how to cope.

Basically I didn't know how to deal with the arbitrary nature of life. No one really teaches you that stuff at school. At least they didn't at mine. My parents tried their best – but how were they supposed to help me navigate my existential conundrums when they were yet to navigate their own?

If I was so consumed by self-doubt and terror, how had I managed to build a life that seemed so fortunate? Because I had Anna.

She is really different from me: she is measured and calm; she is modest and un-showy; she is quietly clever and dryly hilarious. She carries with her none of the doubts or fears or constant needs for reassurance and validation that I was always burdened by (still am a little bit, just a lot less so these days). I have a great deal to thank her parents for. Not just because they have always been so kind to me. But because they raised her with a love, stability and intelligence that I have benefitted from immeasurably. She's got two brothers, Tom and Pete, who I love as if they were my own blood. Joining someone else's family, and forming bonds with all the individuals inside it, is a true privilege.

Anna loves me. And that is really what saved me from pissing my life away on booze, drugs and mayhem. She saw me at my worst but loved me anyway. She convinced me that there was something inside, hidden beneath the inebriated fuckface I had become, worth saving. And because I loved and respected her more than anyone in the world I put my faith in her vision of me.

I grew up with Anna. We met at school when we were eleven but we didn't get together until we were twenty. Throughout our teens we were mates. I just thought she was the absolute best person I'd ever met. We spent incredible times together when we were just kids. On a school trip to Greece in 1991, when we were both sixteen, we snuck out of the hotel one night and went to a local disco. We got absolutely leathered on Blue Curaçao cocktails and, when the DJ dug out 'Step On' by the Happy Mondays, she climbed on my shoulders, we hit the dancefloor and for a moment we were disco superstars. Then my weedy, drunken, teenage legs gave way, we collapsed in a mess and were asked to leave. I knew I loved her even back then.

She was just the best company, all the time. I only ever wanted to hang around with Anna. She was fun, yes. But she was sharp too: clever and occasionally brutal in a way I found somehow intoxicating. Spending time with anyone else was like being short changed by life.

We both did a lot of drinking when we were first together.

Then a moment came where she started tapering off all that stuff. There was no epiphany – it was like her drinking days naturally faded away as she matured and broadened her horizons. She became the sort of person who could easily have one glass of wine with dinner and leave it slightly unfinished.

I thought it was weird. In fact, I found it annoying at times. It even made me angry. I assumed she was judging me. But looking back, I don't think Anna ever judged me for continuing to chuck back lagers or do weekend coke with the lads. She probably just thought, in her own quiet and accepting way, that I was maturing at a slightly slower pace than her and would catch up eventually.

Only I didn't. I allowed my fun drinking to morph stealthily into sleazy, weirdo drinking. She tells me that one of the first warning signs was when I oversaw the kids' bath time with a can of Stella on the go.

Fuck me, that wasn't the half of it.

By this stage, the whole *I'm just a bit of a lad who likes a few beers at the weekend* act was long gone. My tolerance threshold had been driven steadily up over decades of fun-time drinking. I needed an ever-increasing quantity of booze just to achieve the same buzz. This meant I had to drink amounts that would be considered socially unacceptable even in the most liberal of circles. Beers at bath time were one thing but not nearly as scary as the drinking I had started to do in secret.

Miniature vodkas stashed in my office to top me up through the working day. Those secret night-time runs to the bins two streets away to dispose of all my empties. Locking myself in the toilet at polite, afternoon family get-togethers in order to turbo-down the cans of beer I had taken from the fridge and smuggled up my jumper or down my trousers. More often than not chased down with lines of coke. I had to drink at a level of intensity that was just seedy and embarrassing. At least I had enough self-awareness to realise how fucking depressing my behaviour had become.

I came to realise, eventually, that I didn't need to be pitiful.

And I didn't need to be scared.

I could be a good bloke who found happiness and fulfilment in the things that already surrounded me. My wife and my kids could bring me all the joy, all the fun, all the validation I needed. The future might hold a few surprises, yes. But if I was sober I could face anything with clear eyes, a full heart and faith in myself.

More than anything, I just wanted my relationship with Anna back. We had been together since we were twenty and held hands through all of the formative events in our lives. We were in love but we were best mates too. I had soured our whole friendship by effectively having an affair with alcohol. It made me lie. It made me resentful. It made me boring. Why would she want to spend time with a cunt like that?

So I went and got help. Because I knew what the reward was: my life, the one I had already built but had been too thick to appreciate.

Booze is a bastard. It tries to tell you that any time you spend without it is wasted. That all the other things in your life are dreary by comparison. That you can only really be your true self when you are in its company. The reverse is true of all those things, of course. Love is the only thing any of us need. I was wasting my time when I wasn't with the person who loved me most. I wasn't my true self: I was bored and lonely and bitter and confused. When I am with Anna I am happy and confident and at my absolute best.

I am really grateful for my seven years of sobriety. But not half as grateful as I am for Anna. Life gave me one last choice back in 2015 – and I chose love.

19

Thank You, Alcohol

Without booze taking hold of me, kicking my head in, stealing my money and making me a cunt I would never be the person I am today. Which is not to say I am a perfect person. I am just better than I was in June 2015 when I had my last drink. A lot fucking better. Not just because I am no longer hung over and grumpy all the time. Not just because I no longer get lairy and abusive in public. And not just because I no longer sneak about the house stealing swigs of voddy when the kids are in bed and the wife's in a different room.

I am better because once I'd knocked all that stuff on the head I began to ask myself why I had needed to drink and take drugs in the first place. As I've already explained, I realised that I was constantly in search of some external validation to make myself feel happy and secure. Attention, money, respect, success: these are the sort of things I craved. And when I wasn't getting enough of those things I would look for an escape in drugs and booze. Had I not got sober I might never have confronted the real problem: a gaping hole inside. An itch that needed scratching. A generalised dissatisfaction with myself.

Booze had been a sticking plaster for too long. Once I tore it off I was forced to seek longer term, more meaningful solutions to my malaise. I had to learn how to be comfortable with myself and accepting of the shit life throws at us. So, thank you alcohol, I guess. Without you I would never have gone through the painful but rewarding process of getting my crap together. It took me forty years but eventually I started to learn the difference between the important stuff and the bullshit.

I never hit rock bottom. That is to say I never ended up pissing my pants in a budget meeting or getting arrested for public indecency. I didn't lose my home or my family or anything really bad like that.

But like so many alcoholics (I would guess the vast majority) I was locked in a sort of purgatory that was somehow worse. I mean, if I had shat myself or got nicked, at least I'd have a good story to tell when people ask me why I no longer drink.

My drinking started when I was twelve and, at a pace so slow it was almost imperceptible, it grew into an ugly and destructive habit by the time I was in my mid-thirties. By the time I realised it was no longer something I did for fun but something I did to numb pain and discomfort, it was almost too late.

One thing I told myself back then was that my drinking didn't affect anyone else. It was a private decision and an expression of personal freedom. I told myself that I liked drinking and deserved to have things that I liked. But all of that was bollocks. I didn't really like drinking; it had just become learned behaviour because I had been doing it for so long. It started out as something I did to look cool and grown up; then it was just part of the culture that surrounded me so I did it to fit in; sometimes I did it for the courage and confidence I had simply not learned to muster while sober; eventually I was just doing it because I had forgotten how to cope with everyday life without a drink inside me.

I told myself that I was able to compartmentalise my drinking. It's true I would try to not get pissed in front of the kids (but even that rule went out the window on certain occasions such as Christmas Day when, like all pisshead dads, I legitimised guzzling beers and Scotch in front of my children from breakfast through to bedtime).

I told myself that drinking was part of my private time. This meant that I did it with mates at the football or on Friday night or – as my problem got worse – sitting in the corner of a pub on my own all afternoon.

But none of this really protected my loved ones from the impact of my boozing. I was grumpy and tired all the time. My mind was almost always on my last drink or my next drink. I built too many social engagements and even family occasions around getting high. I invited a coke dealer to my mum's seventieth, for fuck's sake (to be fair, he did great business that night).

I was demonstrably shitter at being a dad, a husband, a son, a brother, a mate and a colleague when I was drinking. Anyone who is boozing regularly will be the same, whether they want to admit it to themselves or not. It's hard to make that admission because the booze takes over your mind and tells you it's really not a big deal. *Having a few drinks is normal*, it says. *It's fun. It's your right. It doesn't hurt anyone else.*

Booze is full of shit. With any luck, one day you get a moment of clarity, realise that alcohol has been gaslighting you for years and that, in fact, getting pissed all the time really is a big deal. 'I don't get pissed, I just like a drink,' I would tell people back then. As if my heightened tolerance to alcohol somehow made me healthier.

People talk about the importance of willpower when you are giving up drink. Yes, you need that in the early stages. But you need so much more. Willpower might help you stop drinking for a day, a week, a month or even a year. But you will not stay sober and learn to embrace all of the joys that go with it unless you address the deeper issues. Why did you drink? What is the matter? How do you feel? Why can't you seem to relax? These are tough questions. They might seem a bit overblown. You might think that you drink because it tastes nice or you like the feeling it gives you. But why do you need that feeling? That five-minute buzz followed by an uncomfortable craving followed by gradual anticlimax, then grogginess then nausea then self-hatred and shame. Who needs that shit in their life?

Of course, you might not have a problem with drink, which is great. But everyone has a problem with themselves. Everyone has a nameless worry that's constantly whispering in their ear, trying to get their attention. You might not use booze to cope with it. Maybe you use exercise, spending, sex or Haribos. Or maybe you've got no obvious bad habits but sometimes just feel miserable or bad about yourself in an unspecific way. The problem, I reckon, is that we live in a society that places all the emphasis on externalised solutions to our problems. In the olden times, they had religion or some other form of spirituality. But there came a point where we started to think of ourselves as so clever that we didn't need to reflect on our inner selves any more. All we needed was the rewards of modern life: a good job, a nice house, a flash car; the attention and respect of others; the buzz and excitement of constant sensual stimulation.

Have I learned to stop chasing that shit since I stopped drinking? Have I fuck. You should see the state of my overdraft, mate. I suppose the important thing, though, is that I now realise that those cravings are unhealthy. That I am happier and more content when I can ignore my desire for control and external validation; to let go of shit; and to just like myself a bit more unconditionally. It's a lot easier to do that when booze isn't part of your life.

20

Life Is Tough But You Are Tougher

People used to call me Mr Jam because they thought I was lucky. I can remember how it started. My brother's company threw out a mini-fridge in the process of moving offices and, somehow, it ended up in my possession. I was sixteen years old and still living at home with my mum. In my bedroom I had an IKEA bed sofa. Now, I had a mini-fridge with cans of Foster's stored in it too. Sixteen years old, single with a sofa and a fridge? I was basically Frank Sinatra in his absolute prime. Sophisticated. Mature. Unstoppable.

This was the early nineties when mini-fridges were more glamorous and exclusive than they are today. You couldn't pick them up off eBay for twenty quid. A mini-fridge was the sort of thing you only saw in high-class hotel rooms. In that sense, my brothers were right to label me Mr Jam. I truly did appear to be the luckiest man alive.

The Mr Jam moniker stuck as I got older and entered the world of work. In my twenties, things went pretty well for me: I seemed to glide from one exciting job to another. I went from magazines to newspapers to radio and then TV. All of which galvanised the Mr Jam myth. It might have appeared to outsiders that good fortune just landed in my lap but I felt that talent and graft played a big part too.

I realise now that I was also benefitting massively from being white, male and born in London. I wanted to work in the media and I already lived rent free at my mum's, within a city where all the jobs were. Plus I had been exposed to people who made a living out of being creative. I understood that it was a viable career path. It seemed like a realistic ambition. That alone gave me a huge head start.

I didn't fully acknowledge any of that at the time. I was a council-house kid from a state school who had elbowed his way into an industry that was dominated by privately educated wankers and Oxbridge dickheads. So I must have been the underdog. But it's all about context. I had less than some but a great deal more than others.

But all this good fortune meant that when bad luck was eventually visited upon me I was ill prepared. I quit my job as a magazine editor at thirty-five partly because the job consumed so much of my time and energy that I was unable to be a proper dad to my new baby daughter. I also did it because I had grown tired of having bosses. But what made it easier was that I was inundated with offers of extracurricular work. I couldn't keep up with it all. I worked out that I could earn the same – or maybe even more – as a freelancer than as a full-time magazine editor. Why bust my ass ten hours a day (twelve on press days) and deal with irritating management figures when I could earn the same dough at home, be my own boss and get to read my kid a bedtime story every night? It was a no brainer. I quit.

I had three big projects lined up for my first year back as a freelancer. They were lucrative and exciting. They would allow me to reclaim my life. But guess what? They all just disappeared as quickly as they had arrived. The ill-fated documentary I have already mentioned; the other two just fizzled like these things sometimes do.

Everyone has bad luck from time to time. These days, older and a bit wiser, I tell young freelancers that they should be aiming for a success ratio of one in every five projects they go up for. That's perfectly realistic. But back in those days I was more accustomed to the rather less realistic aim of winning five in every five projects I went up for. So when I tasted three successive rejections in a short space of time – rejections that were massive, completely unexpected and, in my case, totally unprecedented – I almost fell to pieces.

I had blithely walked away from the security of a salary, burning bridges in the process, with the cocky glee of a bloke who'd had a mini-fridge in his bedroom when he was just sixteen. I thought that opportunities would simply continue to present themselves to me for ever and ever. Was it a sense of entitlement? No, I didn't think that I necessarily deserved all the breaks. I was just used to getting all the breaks. But then Lady Fortune sucker-punched me and I found myself on my arse, consumed by dread, panic and plummeting self-esteem. Soon, I was skint. The world seemed to be collapsing around my ears. How would I pay the mortgage? How would I feed my kid? What would everyone say? I felt like Ol' Gil, the crumpled, hapless salesman out of *The Simpsons*.

Now I am deep into my forties. I am still basically a freelancer. I have ups and downs. I have good months where the work and money seem to flow like water. And I have bad months when I struggle to make ends meet. And in the midst of those dry spells I still feel a bit down. I get stressed if a big bill lands. Sometimes my ego feels a bit bruised. But one thing I no longer do is panic. I don't interpret a slow period as a symbol of total and irreversible decline. I don't question my own abilities or worry about how other people perceive me. I don't start planning to sell off the kitchen appliances on eBay. I step back, take a breath, make sure I rest properly and eat well. I exercise. I keep working. I just focus on the next step in front of me.

When the shit seemed to have hit the fan back in my mid-thirties I had not learned these habits. Worse, I had no faith in myself. I was unused to facing adversity. I worried that I didn't have the strength to navigate my way through tough times.

One of the best things about that period was that I went so barmy with anxiety that I was forced to confront the problem, see my GP, get some therapy and start the journey into self-awareness that, ultimately, has led me here – writing this down in the hope it might help others who experience the same sort of shit.

Nowadays when I feel shit at least I have faith it will eventually pass. Anxiety can be harder to combat. But the way I stave it off is simply to recall all the bad stuff I've faced down in the past. As someone clever once said: 'Today is the tomorrow you worried about yesterday.'

I am not saying that everything turns out OK in the end. That is bollocks for corny memes. Shit happens. And sometimes it keeps happening. But when it does, I remind myself of all the other bad times that seemed like they might never end. It gives me belief and courage.

Whoever you are, I know you'll have been through your own stuff. And look at you, you're still standing. Remember that. Think about all the times it has happened in the past. Think of the break ups, the rejections, the financial blows or the career hiccups that have kicked you in the balls. They felt awful at the time. They might have set you back a few steps. But here you are, still standing – probably wiser and definitely stronger. You are a fighter. All the evidence points to that. You have come this far because whenever life knocks you down you get back up and laugh in its face. Life is tough – but you are tougher.

21

Getting Sober Is the Best Fun I've Ever Had

When I was a kid, school holidays felt like a drag. I'd read all those Enid Blyton books about posh kids having adventures and picnics all summer long. I assumed that's what most young people were doing while I was sitting indoors on my own, cowering from the hot sunshine like Gollum, eating chocolate digestives and watching *Crown Court*. It was boring, lonely and miserable.

Oh boo-fucking-hoo. Poor me. I spent summer holidays all lonely and glum. Yes, I now realise that my story was nothing special. Sitting about being bored was what most other kids were probably doing too. Or maybe they weren't? I don't know, I didn't ask. All I know is that my mum had to work so from the age of about twelve I tended to while away those long summer holidays skulking about the house on my own, feeling sorry for myself, too lethargic and unimaginative to get out and about (and that was before I discovered wanking, after which there barely seemed any point in getting out of bed at all).

Sitting about doing sod all really did get me down. I was a bored, lazy and chubby kid who let days, weeks – sometimes months – slip by anonymously, then looked around bewildered when school started up again and my peers all seemed taller, older, wiser, more worldly while I had just got fatter and paler.

As I got older I went completely the other way, developing a fixation with socialising and action to stave off those childhood feelings of inadequacy. It would have been great if I had channelled all of that pent-up energy into fitness, academia or spiritual learning. Instead I ploughed it into hedonistic abuse.

When adulthood approached I ploughed the same amount of excessive energy into work. When I landed my first job in journalism I told myself that the best way to succeed was to never stop. When I finished at the office I would go home and write down ideas, do bits of research, read other newspapers and magazines obsessively. I was a product of Thatcherism – totally in thrall to my own productivity. I didn't just want a steady job that paid the bills. I wanted to create great things constantly and be defined by them. And I also wanted to get totally shitfaced every weekend (plus sometimes on a Thursday).

I rarely rested. I had no interests apart from work and getting on it.

I told myself that football was my hobby. But going to football was always as much about getting twatted as it was watching the game. Similarly, playing Monday-night five-a-side was only a ritual we endured prior to the post-match beers.

I craved stimulation at all times. I was terrified of even fleeting moments of boredom. I thought of myself as being constantly on the run from lapsing into that fat bored kid I had once been. The truth is, I was probably just scared of ever being alone with my own unfiltered thoughts.

I used to worry that getting sober would be boring.

Back then, I had no idea how to have fun or keep myself interested without the distraction of work, drink or drugs. I had never learned how to fill my time up in more wholesome ways. I had never learned how to relax in my own company. I had an extremely narrow worldview. I was about as good at being a human as a baby who only knows how to shit itself, eat and cry.

I wish I'd had some hobbies when I was a kid. If I had, I would have been a better adult. But in the 1980s, 'hobby' was a dirty word. Hobbies were for spods: they played chess or watched birds or collected stamps. Taking up a hobby was a sign of giving up. I would watch those weird kids on *Why Don't You?* telling me how to build things out of shoeboxes and Fairy Liquid bottles and I would pity them. 'Dickheads,' I would say, laughing to myself as I was sitting in my dressing gown munching my third bag of crisps of the morning.

When I finally knocked all the drink and drugs on the head I was bored for about three days.

But, luckily, the boredom was overshadowed by all the anxiety, fatigue and profuse sweating. Once I had white-knuckled it through those initial seventy-two hours, I started to feel energised and excited about a life that was suddenly full of possibilities. I had a ton of energy and acres of time to fill with it. The problem was, I didn't quite know how to fill it.

That was why my first three years of sobriety were the busiest of my life. I trained for and ran a half marathon; I lost a couple of stone; I started my own company, launched my own TV programme, hosted a daily three-hour radio show and took on all sorts of other daft projects – all while trying to plough as much time and energy as I could into raising my kids. I said yes to almost everything. And in the end I crashed. I found myself physically and mentally exhausted. Mercifully, I didn't fall off the wagon but I got close at times. I had a therapist who was there to point out that I was overstretched and overwhelmed, and had simply replaced the hedonism with yet more work and exercise. The mind can only take so much before it starts spilling over.

Eventually, there was a collapse. There always is. Since then, I have rebuilt my life in a simpler way that is easier to manage.

I am still very much a work in progress. I still overdo it sometimes. I still say yes to things I shouldn't. I sometimes fill dead evenings with chocolate and make myself an espresso at 8 p.m. at night because . . . I don't know why – it's just something to do, innit?

But I have hobbies. I really do play chess. I really do have a birdwatching book that I have been known to take to the local wetlands centre with me. I read more than I have ever done. And aside from all of that, I just enjoy the seemingly ordinary stuff that surrounds me every day: from the peculiar activities of the local cats that hang about in my street to the ritual of making myself a pot of tea in the afternoon. I stick records on and try to listen to them without distraction. I put my phone on airplane mode for long stretches of the day. I switch off. Learning to do so has been tough; in some ways, tougher than the initial challenge of stopping drink and drugs.

I have had to train myself not to fear idleness but to embrace it. I have had to discover beauty and fun in the day-to-day. It is all there in front of us. Nora Ephron, the famous Hollywood screenwriter, once said: 'Interesting stories happen to people who know how to tell them'. Nowadays, I spend most of my time telling people stories. Sometimes they ask me how come so many interesting things happen to me. They don't. The same amount of remarkable, funny or stimulating things happen to me as to the next person. It's just that, these days, I am clear-eyed enough to see them.

22

If You Want to Quit Drinking, Pick the Right Role Model

February 1993 was the first time I ever ordered a vodka Martini. I remember it specifically because it was my dad's birthday, and I was at a fancy restaurant with my family. Already half pissed, I crept away from the table where we were sitting and staggered towards the long bar in a separate room. It was buzzing with fashionable customers, staffed by po-faced wankers and adorned with an array of the most colourful and exotic boozes I had ever seen. I was seventeen, lank-haired, gormless and dressed in an oversized suit I had borrowed from my older brother for the occasion. Bleary eyed and full of pissed-up bravado I shoved my way to the front of the crowd and confidently demanded, 'A Martini please – with the olive in it.'

The reason I was specific about the olive was because I didn't want them to think I was after one of the Martini Biancos with lemonade that my mum drank at home on special occasions. I was not well-versed in cocktail menus or flash-bar etiquette.

In fact, the only alcohol I had ever ordered was pints of lager in one of the handful of pubs in my area that were willing to serve adolescents in the early nineties. I was therefore surprised when the moody barman started assembling the drink without asking me for any proof of age.

Fuck me, I've pulled it off, I thought to myself. *Look at me, ordering Martinis at fancy bars up west! I am so urbane! I bet all the sexy older women in this place fancy the bollocks off me!*

The barman placed the drink in front of me in that silly triangular glass they come in and I blithely told him to stick it on the bill of our table. Then I felt a hand on my shoulder and turned to see Theo stood behind me, grinning.

'What's all this?' he asked.

'I'm just having a drink, aren't I?' I replied.

'Oh yeah, what drink?'

I hesitated. I stuttered. And then I lied.

'Just . . . a beer.'

'That's not a beer, is it?' he laughed, pointing at the daft concoction sitting on the bar in front of me. 'That's a fucking Martini!'

Before I knew what was happening, he was beckoning my other two brothers over to witness what was happening.

'Come and look at this! Sam has ordered a Martini! With a fucking olive in it!'

The three of them crowded round me, forming a circle and laughing. They prodded and shoved me a bit, then passed the drink around among themselves, pointing their noses in the air and saying things like: 'Pardon me, may I order one of your finest Martinis please, barperson?' in silly posh voices.

Everyone else at the bar, including the attractive older women I had just moments beforehand been contemplating as possible sexual partners, stopped and looked at me. And they began to laugh. So I did what any other self-respecting seventeen-year-old in an oversized suit who had just been caught by his older siblings ordering a vodka Martini in a fancy bar would do: I shouted, 'FUCK OFF!' at them and stormed out of the restaurant.

I do not write any of this expecting sympathy. My brothers were right to bully me that night. And the onlookers were right to laugh. Martinis are stupid drinks: they look daft and they taste disgusting. Even in 1993 they cost about ten quid a pop. Anyone ordering one would look like a bit of a wanker – but a gauche adolescent even more so.

I need hardly tell you why I had ordered it: I had recently watched a James Bond film. In the films, you can easily get wrapped up in Bond's universe of natty suits, fast cars and dreadful chat-up lines. If you're an idiot seventeen-year-old you can go as far as to think you could actually live like Bond, even though you have no money or driving licence and have only ever fingered two girls.

The closest you can get to tasting even a bit of Bond's seemingly glamorous (but, let's be honest, fucking weird) lifestyle is ordering his favourite drink. Booze in Bond films seems so sumptuous, so beautiful, so free of consequence. Bond can drive, fight and fuck like an absolute pro even with a couple of bottles of vodka inside him. And he never gets hangovers or ill-advisedly buys a Big Mac to eat on the way home.

That was the first but not the last case of me trying to take on an aspirational drinking persona. Throughout my drinking years I tried out dozens of them. When I wasn't fantasising about being a ritzy cocktail man I was being a hard-bitten whisky drinker, slumped at a bar with a large Johnnie Walker as if I was just back from saving a village of Mexican peasants from unscrupulous gold prospectors.

A lot of the time I was a lager-smashing, gak-snorting yob, shouting 'Oi oi!' at no one in particular, for no discernible reason, in public places. Sometimes I was a mysterious executive like Don Draper, nursing a drink and wrestling with exotic demons in the corner of a bar. As I reached middle-aged fatherhood I would sometimes like to play the wine expert, blowing stupid sums of money on bottles of drink I didn't really understand or particularly like in upmarket booze emporiums where I would spend ages talking to the salesperson like a big, deluded ponce.

Sometimes I was Jerry out of *The Good Life*: coming home from a hard day at the office and immediately pouring myself a large glass of something amber and strong, letting out a loud sigh of decompression as the strains of the day melted into boozy oblivion.

But whoever I was trying to be, whatever drink I was drinking and wherever I was doing it, I was still the same pathetic fantasist I had been at that bar in February 1993.

I was still trying to see myself through the prism of something I had digested on TV or in a movie. I was like a pissed-up Mr Benn, trying out different roles, each of them as removed from the reality of my life as the next. All to feel comfortable with myself.

There is so much delusion in boozing.

When you're a kid you think it makes you cool. By the time you've grown out of that, you're semi-hooked on the stuff so you have to create fantasies to justify your drinking. So you create a vision of yourself as a cosy old-man drinker or a good-times party-guy drinker or a mad hooligan drinker or refined wine-shop drinker. But it's all just booze, it just comes in different colours and different bottles to trick you. Most of it is a marketing scam, invented by people who know all about the little stories we tell ourselves and have clever ways of exploiting them. They create myths around drink: the mysterious cowboy; the saloon bar hardman; the poncy spy with the Aston Martin and the rampant misogyny issues.

To help me give up boozing I didn't stop telling myself stories; I just tried to tell better ones.

First, I looked around me to see who I knew that didn't drink at all. There were three or four blokes, all older than me, that I had socialised with for years who never touched a drop. They were not boring or pious or preachy. They were fun and relaxed and – in every case – pretty successful too. They were fun to be around but rarely lost control. There was something about the fact they didn't drink that made them seem appealingly confident.

I realised that these were the sort of people I wanted to be like. Meanwhile, I looked at the people who were five, ten or twenty years older than me and still going hard at it – and I felt sick at the thought of turning out like them.

One day I googled 'famous people who don't drink' and was surprised by some of the names on the list. Many of them were reformed addicts who, often, had seen a huge upturn in their professional and personal fortunes once they had knocked the booze on the head. But others were just people who had never chosen to drink in the first place. Prince, my all-time favourite musician, was one. Another was Chuck D from Public Enemy, a man I've always thought is the coolest person on earth. Chuck D is creative, pioneering, wildly clever, passionate, militant, well dressed and, while not a man of violence, would probably be handy in a tear up if he was forced into a corner. He is not the boring, vanilla sort of non-drinker that lived inside my younger mind.

I am a white, middle-aged dad who lives in leafy south-west London and enjoys long walks, scented candles and looking at cats. I will never be Chuck D. But I am happy and comforted to know that we share at least one thing in common: neither of us wants to be fucking James Bond.

23

The Big Secret about
Giving Up Booze

They call it the 'pink cloud' – a sudden feeling of euphoria that
hits you about a month or so after you quit booze and drugs.
All the last traces of your bad habits finally leave your body and –
WHOOSH – you start seeing the world through new eyes. Yeah,
I thought it was bullshit too. But, turns out, it's very real.

I was on a train on the way back from a work trip to
Yorkshire when it first hit me. Rattling through the countryside
at high speed, watching sheep blur past on the sun-dappled
hillsides, I suddenly got an overwhelming sense of wonder and
joy. It was strange. I was not drunk, I was not high. I was not
having sex or watching *Return of the Jedi*. None of my usual joy
triggers was at play. I was just sitting on my arse, minding my
own business, looking out of a window at some sheep. And I
felt absolutely brilliant.

Don't worry, this isn't the bit where I tell you that I turned
to see Jesus Christ sitting next to me right there in second class,

smiling benignly and telling me that my sinful life was at an end. It was just that my brain had finally managed to expunge the last traces of the crap I'd been filling it with for the past twenty-five years. It was like a dried up old mushroom that had suddenly been rehydrated.

In the days and weeks that followed, the feeling hung around. I began to take pleasure in the everyday. Air smelt fresher, leaves looked greener, crisps tasted . . . crispier. I realised that these everyday pleasures had always been there but, for the most part, my drunken brain had been too distracted to properly appreciate them.

I'm not saying I had been perma-pissed for the past twenty-five years. But I had built a lifestyle where drinks were always hovering about somewhere in my mind. Either I was about to get drunk, actually in the state of being drunk, thinking about a future time in which I would be drunk, regretting a time when I had been excessively drunk or just promising myself that I would never, ever get drunk again. Having those sorts of booze thoughts constantly humming away in the back of your mind is exhausting and boring too.

Once I made the unilateral decision to stop drinking permanently, all that bullshit was lifted away. The tedious rules I made up (and loudly bored everyone around me with) about when and how I drank were suddenly redundant. I could stop pretending to myself that being inebriation-free for three days a week made me strong-willed and superior.

The pink cloud made me feel both calm and excited. I felt tingly optimism but without the nervous energy that usually came with it. In the past, I had struggled to harness feelings of joy without them spilling over into a manic anxiety that I would seek to defuse with booze and drugs. If West Ham won a big match my only response was to get shitfaced. It would stop my mind from spinning. Looking back, it was a shame: I squandered natural happiness by smothering it in alcohol. Which is doubly wasteful when you think about how rarely West Ham win.

The instinct to drink at times of joy is partly cultural: we've been trained by adverts and TV to think that you're not really honouring a happy moment unless you're guzzling booze. But I think it is also biological: happiness can sometimes feel a bit too much to cope with. Your mind can go into overdrive, your heart can beat faster, you just don't know what to do with yourself.

The pink cloud allowed me to just ride the wave of contentment without it getting out of hand. The closest narcotic buzz I could compare it to is being high on weed – but without the paranoia, snackiness or lethargy.

I received a phone call one sunny afternoon in August, telling me that I had landed a job producing and presenting my own TV series. It was the first time since getting sober that I had received major, exciting news. Every instinct told me that the only way to mark the occasion was to get pissed. But I really didn't want to. I just couldn't think of what else to do – a lifetime of booze and drugs can make you profoundly unimaginative.

In the end, I walked up the street to an ice-cream shop, bought myself a double cone and sat on a wall, the sun on my face, luxuriating like a cat on a shed roof. And for the first time since I was about twelve, I just lived in the moment. I've been trying my best to do the same ever since.

The thing about the pink cloud is that it doesn't last. The initial rush of sober euphoria fades like everything else does and soon you are confronted with all the irritating concerns and worries of ordinary life. You can't just surf over them using the superpower of sobriety for ever. You realise that life's problems and anxieties can never be eradicated completely. All you can do is start to work out ways of coping that don't involve booze. Learning to do that is something you might work on every day and never fully master. But that doesn't matter. It's all about progress, not perfection.

24

What I Tell Young People about Booze and Drugs

When I first started going out at weekends with my mates, I would be nervous about booze and drugs. Some of the other kids were much more cavalier than me. But I didn't want to feel left out so I would ignore the voices in my head telling me to be cautious and just crack on with stuff. I don't regret it that much. I mean, nothing bad came of it for any of us. Other than the subsequent thirty years of lost nights, incidents of mayhem and embarrassment, stupidity, illness, conflict, expense, broken relationships, shame and deep sadness.

Loads of my mates have had dependency issues with drugs or alcohol over the years. And many of us have struggled with depression at some stage (yeah, you should come hang out with us some time, we're a right barrel of laughs). Of course, we might well have all hit a brick wall of stress and existential panic in middle age either way. At least we had fun getting off our faces together when we were younger, the hangovers weren't as bad and we seemed to have an infinite supply of get-out-of-jail-free cards.

Younger blokes have asked me if it is wise for them to 'get it out of their system' while they're still able to live with relatively few responsibilities. As a former pisshead turned slightly weird sobriety evangelist, I try my best not to be too preachy (if I'm failing, sue me). So I usually say, 'Yeah, go for it, squeeze it all in now before you have to start getting up at 5 a.m. to change shitty nappies, mate.'

But that's just more of my bullshit. It suggests that I still regard booze and drugs as desirable lifestyle choices – just ones I have had to forgo because I let them get out of hand. I don't. I regard them as a waste of time. A large part of me wishes I'd never got into any of that stuff in the first place. Yes, I had some good times while off my nut. Dancing, partying, laughing, being stupid, doing and saying things I might not have had the balls to do or say had I been sober. But in all of those happy memories drugs and alcohol merely played the role of facilitator. They gave me the courage and sense of abandon I required to create and relish those moments.

What I wish is that I'd had the bollocks to experience those moments naturally. To have danced and laughed and been stupid and all that other shit just because I wanted to do it, knew it was fun and didn't really give a fuck what anyone else thought of me.

That's what I'm like now. I am stupid all the time. I laugh all the time. I wouldn't say I dance all the time – but I probably dance about as much as I ever did (roughly three to four times a week, mostly in the kitchen, if you're wondering). Mind you, that's not because I have reached a state of sober enlightenment. It's just because I'm an embarrassing forty-seven-year-old dad who's given up on the idea of dignity.

The point is that booze and drugs weren't ever the things that made my life fun.

They were just the things that fast-tracked me to experiencing that fun without the self-consciousness that sometimes held me back. But I am now a grown-up so can do those things without stabilisers.

I hope my kids develop a wider worldview than the one with which I grew up.

I hope they will see booze as something that's a nice occasional treat – like a Mars bar – rather than a lifestyle choice. That way, they won't be asking me when they're in their twenties if it's important to continually get spannered after work in order to 'get it out of the system'. Enjoying life is not something you need to get out of your system. But relying on booze and drugs to do so probably is.

25

My Ego, the Bastard

It was Malta in the final days of summer 2017. I was miserable, knackered and didn't want to be there. To make matters worse, when I got to my hotel room, desperate for a shower and a kip, it stank of piss.

I got on the blower to reception. 'Sorry to bother you but my room stinks of piss. Can I get a different one?'

'What kind of room do you want, Mr Delaney?'

'Ideally one that doesn't stink of piss, please.'

They said they'd see what they could do. I waited twenty minutes and, having heard nothing back from my hosts, I checked out and found somewhere round the corner that was slightly less disgusting.

Looking back on that depressing trip I realise that the hotel room stank of piss for a reason.

I shouldn't have been in Malta and the universe knew it. The universe made sure I wound up in that piss-stinking room as a means of telling me: 'Get the fuck out of there, Sam. Jump on a plane home. This is not what you should be doing with your life.'

The universe was, as always, dead right.

I was in Malta for work. Work that I had no interest in. Work that was truly toxic – not just for me but for society at large.

I was with some colleagues in pursuit of some business as 'content creators' for a dreary commercial client.

Awful people in crappy suits refer to this sort of thing as 'content marketing'. It was a field I had stumbled into by mistake, having started my own entertainment company a few years previously to make fun TV and radio shows. I just wanted to earn a living by making the sort of daft stuff I liked to watch or listen to. But a couple of years down the line, here I was selling myself out to a bunch of tedious businessmen in awful suits.

Granted, I knew less about the evils of the gambling industry then than I do now. Through meeting recovering gamblers, I have gained insight to the insidious and malignant ways in which these companies actually cultivate and nurture addiction – and how that addiction wrecks (and sometimes ends) thousands of lives in the UK every year.

Back then, I didn't know the stats. But I can't really use ignorance as my defence. I mean, we all know there's something a bit iffy about these outfits, don't we? I'm not judging anyone who likes a flutter. But I am judging myself for getting into bed with an industry that has prominent red flags all over it.

On reflection, I can see what was happening in my life at that time. I had got sober in 2015 and, over the next two years, as if the universe was rewarding me, my business had sky-rocketed. The work didn't seem to stop coming in. And most of it was great fun – work I enjoyed doing and felt proud of.

But soon other jobs started coming my way that I should have known instinctively were a bad fit. My brother Theo once taught me a helpful system for selecting what jobs to work on. He said you should only ever pick a job if it ticked at least two out of these three boxes: 1. Is it a laugh? 2. Will it further my career? 3. Is the money decent? It had always worked for me before. I'd go as far as to say it is a failsafe system. But in 2017 my ego had taken over and I had stopped using it. I was only focusing on the third box. Money had become a dangerous preoccupation.

The Maltese job wasn't aligned with what was right for me mentally, physically or spiritually. To put it bluntly, the money was great but it was a shit job that would make me feel like a cunt about myself. On top of that, it necessitated me flying off to Malta to give a presentation to people I didn't like about a subject I didn't care about. This was everything I had tried to avoid in my career. I was listening to the wrong people and living up to all the wrong expectations. My head had been turned.

We got that business, and the company made some money from it, but within six months everything was collapsing. Not just the company but me too. Mentally and physically I was fucked. By 2018, I was begging the doctor to up my medication, asking my therapist if she would see me three times a week, talking to my wife every day about how I just couldn't cope any more. I now realise that my mini-breakdown had to happen. I was in the wrong game and I had to get out.

I had burned out. The very simple cause of this was that I had said yes to everyone and everything for too long. Maybe I thought that my sobriety had given me a superpower that allowed me to fit more than twenty-four hours into a single day. But really, I had just had my head turned by success, growth and money as an end in itself. I had forgotten what I really wanted out of my life.

213

I would get better eventually. But first I had to go through some major challenges that would put my sobriety and my sanity to the test.

26

How a Podcast Saved My Life

I think it was Oscar Wilde who said, 'To lose one job might be counted as unfortunate but to lose two in the space of a month must be a fucking nightmare, mate.'

And he wasn't wrong. I should know, it happened to me back in 2018. For the past few years I had been jogging along very nicely, with my own daily radio show and weekly TV programme.

All gigs come to an end eventually. The trick is not to take it personally, move on quickly and always have a Plan B up your sleeve (sometimes Plans C, D and E come in handy too).

But in the spring of 2018 everything came crashing down all at once in a way I just wasn't prepared for.

I was told my radio contract wouldn't be renewed. To be honest, I had seen that coming, was grateful for the two-year run I'd had and was pretty much ready to jack it in anyway. Presenting a daily news and politics show has a natural lifespan. It drives you mad. There are some people who have done it for years – I regard them as superhuman. My show had given me the chance to cover general elections at Westminster, the whole Brexit campaign and even the 2016 presidential elections, which included a week in Washington. I had been able to pivot into political journalism for a few years, which had been a brilliant experience. I was grateful to the people who had given me the chance to do it. Ultimately, they needed someone more famous than me to help them build the profile of the station. Objectively, I could see it was the right decision.

And at least I still had my TV show to help pay the bills. Only I didn't. Because within a fortnight the TV show would come to an end too. Again, I would have been OK with this in isolation (I was fed up with making the show for all sorts of reasons) but it clearly wasn't ideal timing. But then I still had my production company ticking away in the background, with an office full of busy staffers and trusted lieutenants building a little empire for me to rely on. Only, turns out, I didn't really have that either.

The company had somehow been losing money, despite being almost permanently busy. Plus we owed people money. It was an absolute shit-show. Soon all the busy people in my office were gone and I was sitting in an empty room surrounded by bills wondering what the fuck had just happened.

Suffice to say, I didn't get much sleep that summer. I spent 50 per cent of every night staring at a dark ceiling, breathing unsteadily and wondering whether I could convince my wife and kids to move with me to Denmark (I don't know why I thought Denmark was the solution – they just seem to be so bloody nice out there).

In the past I would have most probably leaned heavily on booze and drugs to help my mind deal with the sudden onslaught of stress and anxiety. But I was pretty confident that I wouldn't relapse: however bad things felt, I remained acutely aware that going back to my addictions would make everything infinitely worse.

I might not have been actually drinking or taking drugs but I wasn't really sober in the purest sense of the word. Since knocking my bad habits on the head in 2015, I had been so busy with work that I hadn't really focused properly on my recovery. They call people like me 'dry drunks'. Just because I had managed to stop filling my body with toxic substances I thought I was better. But shovelling that shit into your system is only ever a symptom of a bigger problem. You don't get into habits that destructive unless there are some deeper, darker feelings lurking behind them.

The sequence of unfortunate events in 2018 forced me to take my recovery a bit more seriously.

I felt simultaneously miserable and frantic. My mind buzzed morning, noon and night with a thousand and one problems – some real, some imaginary. I started chasing work I didn't really want. I filled up my time with nonsense schemes and wild goose chases that I thought might help get me out of the hole I was in. I became too intense.

And then I slowly started to embrace the idea that less was more: that in times of flux or uncertainty, it's usually better to not speed up but slow down. I needed to take it easy, get some rest, allow my mind to process what the fuck was going on in my life and plan my next move in a sober and rational way. Grabbing at possibilities or half chances never works out well. In the worst-case scenarios, you manage to make one of your more frantic, far-out plans come to fruition – and then you're stuck with it. By the time you get sane again it's too late, you're already balls deep in that gravel business you accidentally started in the midst of a mini-breakdown. (Yes, this was genuinely one of the ideas I toyed with when things got bad. Thank God I've got a sensible wife who isn't afraid to tell me to shut the fuck up when I come out with this sort of bollocks.)

One day, in the middle of all this crap, I got an email from my old cohort Andy Dawson asking me if I wanted to do a podcast with him about football nostalgia.

I liked Andy, he made me laugh. I thought just hanging out with him for one hour a week to talk shit might serve as a welcome respite for my troubled mind. I never thought it would be my salvation.

But it was. Not only did it offer a weekly opportunity to just relax into being a dickhead (something which I am excellent at), it started to attract a decent audience and make us a few quid. Which meant I was able to take a more measured and strategic approach to fixing my business. I didn't have to make mad, knee-jerk decisions or barmy, backs-to-the-wall gambles. I had money to pay the bills. I gradually started to navigate the company out of trouble. Slowly, things began to work themselves out.

Just as important was the time I spent looking after myself, resting, reading and learning more about recovery. I realised that stopping drink and drugs was just the very start.

I am so much better now because I balance my life carefully. I already had a great therapist who helped me loads. I also went to see a psychiatrist who, after hearing the story of the last few years of my life, ventured: 'Sounds to me like you've just created space for your next project.' I remember thinking: *What a load of bollocks. Doesn't he realise my life is fucked?* But it turned out he was 100 per cent right. I had ditched a load of stressful unfulfilling stuff and created space for what became the best job I've had in my life. Although doing a podcast isn't really a job, of course. Which is precisely why it is so great.

Lockdown was easier for me than most, not least because I was able to work from home. The increased time spent with my family, away from the more stressful elements of work life, did nothing but good for my mental health. And my experience of recovery gave me the tools I needed to combat the more existential conundrums presented by the pandemic. Accept the things you can control and learn how to tell the difference – that thinking came in very handy throughout 2020. Recovering addicts had a secret advantage during COVID's scariest times.

Change is always a bastard. It's good to recognise that. Sometimes, even seemingly trivial alterations to your usual routine can knock you slightly off track. When they do, it's important to slow down and give yourself a break. Things tend to work out in the end. And you never know what good stuff might be waiting for you round the corner.

The *Top Flight Time Machine* podcast started out as just an amusing distraction but it ended up helping me out of a bad place.

Not just because it's fun and provided me with an income. But because there is a community of like-minded people that has grown around it. It's no longer about football. It's about all sorts of bollocks. But it is also quite honest and sincere, and working with Andy brings out the best in me. I like sharing bits about myself on the podcast and feeling like it connects with listeners. Actually, that sounds a bit wanky. What I really mean is, there are fans who praise us on Twitter, which really panders to my not insubstantial ego. Hey, I said I was in recovery – I never said I was fucking Buddha.

Anyway, thank God Andy emailed me when he did or I might be running a gravel business by now. My point is, salvation can come from the most unexpected places. If you remain calm in a time of crisis, the universe has got a way of intervening and taking care of stuff for you. Just take a breath.

27

How to Help Other People
Without Driving Yourself Mad

My dad, who is in his eighties and lives alone, was feeling a bit under the weather. He'd got a non-COVID chest complaint. When I heard about this I immediately gave him a buzz. As soon as he answered the phone, I started firing frantic questions at him and offering up unsolicited advice. He sounded annoyed by this – which was understandable because it *was* annoying.

For starters, it was the first time I had rung him in ages and the implication was that I could only be bothered making contact with him when there was a chance he might be dying. Plus I was fussing over him like an overbearing parent. My dad is an intelligent adult who knows how to look after himself. Like most adults, he doesn't take kindly to being pitied or patronised. He didn't need or want his youngest son on the blower speaking loudly about chest X-rays and GP referrals like he was a confused child. Thankfully, I realised I was being a dick quite early in the conversation, established that he wasn't actually dying just yet and changed the subject to more enjoyable things, like how much he hates José Mourinho.

I have to be honest: my call was only partly motivated by compassion.

It owed just as much to my own selfish fears. The fear that something bad might happen to my dad, which in turn would impact on my own feelings. I was also motivated by the misplaced belief that I was able to intervene and fix the situation. But what the fuck do I know about lungs?

It's a control issue that is common to lots of people. A desire for control – and the underlying knowledge that I had none – was maybe one of the reasons I used to get pissed all the time. It is dangerous to think that you can create a protective bubble for yourself or your loved ones. We are all subject to the same slings and arrows of life. It doesn't matter if you reckon you're more intelligent, more resourceful or even more rich than the next bloke – sooner or later, someone you love is going to get a chest infection. Shit happens. Get used to it. And have a little faith in the ability of yourself and others to cope.

Life is arbitrary.

You really could be hit by a bus tomorrow. But you probably won't be. You're a grown-up. You will know what action to take. You've dealt with shit before and you will do it again. Things are rarely as bad as they seem. And all of this applies to the people you care about too.

None of us has that much control. There are just too many random factors out there. Getting on with life one day at a time and training yourself not to waste precious headspace on thinking about worst-case scenarios are critical to living a happy, relaxed, relatively sane life. But it's not just your own mad, booby-trapped existence you have to be at peace with.

It's other people's too. There are so many people you care about who are running around living their own lives every day, facing all the same risks and pitfalls that we all face, jeopardising their safety, health and happiness as they do so. If you spend too much time contemplating all of that, you will only succeed in sending yourself bananas.

I have been there many times.

In the past I might have carried on hassling my dad with calls and texts, chasing him up about seeking doctor's appointments or fretting about the tiny fluctuations in his breathing patterns. But not only would that annoy him, it would stress me out for no reason. Having every last piece of information about a situation doesn't make you any more capable of controlling it. My dad doesn't need me to save him. He doesn't need me to guide him through every minor bump in the road. And, even if he did, it is unlikely that I would be able to fix all of his problems anyway. I would just load more and more pressure on to myself – and, like anyone else, I've got enough on my plate as it is.

I hope this doesn't come across like a manifesto for not giving a shit about other people. Yes, it's important to let others know you are there for them. But there is a fine line between being the sort of person others know they can count on in a crisis, and the sort of person who is just a nosey pain in the arse.

Over the years I have tried to implicate myself in the problems of numerous friends and relatives.

Sometimes I have helped, sometimes I haven't. But in every case I have always ended up sharing the stress and concern (sometimes even the financial problems) of those people. Effectively, I have turned one problem into two in the mistaken belief that if I worry on their behalf it will lessen their burden. It never does. I just end up as anxious as they are.

These days I try to let it be known that I am there for mates if they need to get stuff off their chest. And I am open about my own vulnerabilities in the hope it encourages them to do the same, should they need to.

Lastly (and this is one I still struggle with) I will try not to fix things. Instead, I will just listen and try to show understanding. I am not the mental health SAS. I cannot parachute into other people's lives and take their problems away. And even if I could, it wouldn't do them a whole lot of good in the long term.

So now, I prefer to keep my message to others fairly simple:

'I am your mate. I am fucking mental. There is nothing you can tell me about what is going on in your head that I will judge you for. I can't fix things for you. But just talking to me about stuff might help. And if you need a lift to the hospital, I'm your man.'

28

How to Ditch a Dickhead

There is a Buddhist saying that goes: 'Before you speak, let your words pass through three gates: is it true? Is it necessary? Is it kind?'

It's such beautiful guidance; so powerful in its simplicity.

That said, sometimes in life you just really need to call a cunt a cunt.

I have worked hard to be a better, more forgiving and understanding person over the past few years. I am happier and more at peace with myself when I manage to ignore the flaws and foibles of other people, and silently float above unkind words or unfair actions.

But if you really want to stay sane you also need to learn how, when and where to draw the line with toxic people.

I had to do it recently with a bloke I've known for years. He began to offer me unsolicited opinions on my sobriety. I felt it was snide and niggly. People do this sometimes. They feel uncomfortable with your sobriety. Maybe they feel judged or intimidated by it. But they will question you about it to try and cast doubt on its validity. I've got a relative who constantly asks me if I still take drugs, despite the fact he knows I have been very publicly drug free for several years now. It's his way of belittling my sobriety; of indicating I'm just going through a phase. God knows what he personally gets out of this. I'd like to say it doesn't bother me but it really does.

Anyway, this bloke was doing something similar while we were on holiday. He was questioning the fact I had consumed an alcohol-free beer (something strict AA people discourage but I have no problem with). He wouldn't leave the subject alone. I felt as if he was trying to suggest my sobriety was in some way contrived. That I was a fake. I couldn't understand why he was doing it. I was hurt. Maybe I am too sensitive. But my sobriety is important to me. I don't need other people to agree with my choices; I don't even need them to take my problems seriously. I don't want sympathy – but I don't want crafty digs or condescending advice that I didn't ask for, either.

We, particularly the British, are raised to put up and shut up with other people's bullshit in the name of good manners. But sometimes good manners are an excuse to hide behind when you don't have the bollocks to call people out on their behaviour. If someone is fucking with you, you really do have to tell them to stop. Or they will carry on without consequence – making you and everyone else around them miserable. This bloke had been doing it to me – and other people I care about – for years. The jibes about my sobriety were the straw that broke the camel's back.

So I called him out on it. Passive-aggressive people never expect a confrontation – but sometimes you need to give it to them. They squirm under the glare of unexpected scrutiny. I found the confrontation very cathartic.

* * *

Calling a cunt a cunt is spiritually cleansing. That powerful feeling of not letting shit slide is incredible. You tell someone they are being out of order – that they are hurtful and unkind, and that you're not going to take it any more – and all the bitterness and resentment that you might otherwise have carried around inside your stomach for years is gone. You are free: both of those feelings and the dickhead that tried to put them inside you.

Yes, try to avoid rows and arguments whenever possible. But do not be so tolerant that you endanger your own mental health. Look for patterns of toxic behaviour. There is no room for people who consistently try to manipulate you – or those with a record of saying stuff that makes you feel bad.

I know most mental health advice is to avoid anger at all costs. For what it's worth, I don't agree. Anger has its place if you can harness it properly. Sometimes people take the piss. They use up your time and energy – or they try to undermine you in order to soothe their own insecurities. Sometimes we can indulge these people in the name of being selfless. Like most people, I was raised to believe that selfishness is the ultimate sin. This might have made me a bit too eager to please at times. But if you're always trying to please other people and are too scared to ever rock the boat, you end up carrying around resentment. You secretly feel exploited, unappreciated, or even bullied. You might start to feel sorry for yourself.

I used to feel this way sometimes. I was choosing to carry around those sorts of toxic feelings, which would occasionally bubble over at random and inappropriate moments. It would have been much better to have felt a little bit of righteous anger towards the people who made me feel like shit and called them out on it at the time. It's a cleaner way of dealing with problems: to see them, feel them and address them quickly so you can move on.

I have smiled off so many mean and cutting remarks in my life that I still carry with me today. Sometimes they still wake me in the night and force me to rake over stuff that happened decades ago. What a waste of time. I wish that I had never smiled stuff off. I wish I had told those people that they were being mean at the time. I wouldn't have necessarily required an apology from them. Just telling them how I felt would have been cathartic enough. I wouldn't have let them get away with what they probably knew was a fucking liberty.

Sure, Buddhism is great. Yes, we all need to try to understand each other's struggles. But sometimes it's OK to say: 'I forgive you, I understand you, I know you have faced your own challenges . . . but, seriously, get the fuck out of my life.'

Namaste.

29

Life Is about Just One Thing

'You know what the secret of life is? One thing . . . You stick to that and everything else don't mean shit.'

'That's great, but what's the one thing?'

'That's what you've gotta figure out.'

This exchange, from the 1991 movie *City Slickers*, used to frustrate the shit out of me when I was younger. The bloke dishing out the cryptic advice is Curly, a gnarled old cowboy played by Jack Palance. The bloke he's dishing it out to is Mitch, a city-dwelling ponce in the throes of a midlife crisis, played by Billy Crystal.

I was sixteen when *City Slickers* came out and just beginning to dabble in life's big questions.

Of course, I was being pretty half-hearted about it – rather than try to work out the meaning of our existence via the great philosophers or religions I was just trying to pick up what I could from watching comedy westerns. And even then, I wasn't really prepared to make much of an effort. I just wanted Curly to spell out, in layman's terms, why we were here and what we were supposed to be doing. I was like: 'Fuck's sake, Curly, stop being so mysterious and just reveal the key to happiness, you cowboy bastard!'

But since then, having undergone my own mid-life crisis and all sorts of other bewildering bullshit, I have tried a bit harder to work out what Curly was on about. I think he was right. You need to find a type of life that makes sense to you and just stick to it, appreciate it and try to live it the best you can. Life can be lived in a billion different ways. If you are lucky enough to be living in the privileged Western world in the twenty-first century the choices can sometimes be overwhelming. We are surrounded by an array of designs for life – often force fed to us by mass marketing or just subtly promoted by our friends and neighbours.

If you are greedy you will try to live several different lives all at once.

You might be a weekend hooligan and a midweek intellectual. You might be a superdad by day and a drunken fuck-up by night. You might profess to want the simple life but actively pursue the egotistical buzz of the limelight. It's normal. All of these different types of life have their attraction. But ultimately you can only choose one. Trying to juggle them all at once leaves you exhausted, confused and riddled with the ever-present sense that you might be bullshitting yourself and everyone around you.

Curly was a cowboy. He liked driving cattle, eating beans, lassoing stuff and all the other things cowboys do. So he devoted his life to cowboying and loved every minute of it. But Mitch was some sort of busy metropolitan executive who had made all the money and achieved the status he set out for but still found himself feeling a bit empty. He thought playing cowboys might help him discover a new approach to living that would miraculously scratch his itch. But he discovered that it takes more than riding around on a horse in a daft hat to absolve him of his existential malaise.

During lockdown I became increasingly frustrated with the house I live in.

My family and I spent so long inside the same four walls that they started to feel like they were closing in on us. I found myself going berserk over little domestic inconveniences, like the way everything falls out of the Tupperware cupboard every time I open it. Why do we even have so much Tupperware? The bathroom is too small. The hallway is full of coats and shoes and bags. I can't get the vacuum cleaner out from the cupboard under the stairs very easily. Often, I lose my cool about these trivial matters and announce that we need to move house.

I spend hours trawling Rightmove for large homes outside the city with big gardens and plentiful storage space for Tupperware and whatnot. I fantasise about living in a home so spacious that the vacuum cleaner could have an entire room of its own. I go as far as researching local schools in towns I have barely even heard of and tell my wife exactly how we would travel to visit her mum if we were to move out.

But my wife says: 'Shut up, you twat, we're not moving. We love it here, the kids don't need the disruption and you're just going stir crazy. Instead of spending hours staring at houses on your phone, try tidying the kitchen cupboards up a bit so you don't end up going fucking bananas every time you open them.'

Like Curly, she knows the secret of life is just one thing. I'm lucky enough to have found mine: a family I love and a home I was perfectly OK with before a killer virus locked us all inside it for fourteen months.

I don't need to change my reality, I just sometimes need to adjust my perspective on it. Looking at Rightmove is a distraction from the life I am living. It is a way of tricking my brain into believing it wants and needs more to be satisfied. But once I deleted the app from my phone a few weeks ago, tidied the cupboards, organised the hallway and made plans to decorate the bathroom, my psyche settled back down again. I have reminded myself to be grateful for all the things I have and take pleasure in them every day. I try not to constantly look at the horizon or ask what's next. I do my best to relish what's going on right now.

It's like a form of mindfulness – but without all the bullshit mantras and meditation. It's just a matter of staying focused on the things you love about the life you are already living. I saw a sweatshirt the other day emblazoned with a slogan that put it perfectly: 'Remember when you wanted all the things you currently have?'

30

How I Built My Sanity Squad

The year 2014 was probably my darkest ever. I had really allowed myself to fall into a bad place with the drinking and the gear.

I went to my mum's empty cottage on the Isle of Wight one weekend to finish a book I was writing. I was way past my deadline and the publisher was getting jittery. I stared at a blank page for about an hour after I got there, then I just slammed the laptop shut, went to the local Londis, bought a load of cans and a bottle of whisky and wasted the whole weekend boozing, alone.

Eventually I got sober.

One of the best things about my life today is that I do socialise, I have good friends around me, I like myself and (I am pretty sure) my wife likes me too. So do my kids. I am happy and (most of the time) easier to be around. I don't have any drug dealers' numbers in my phone and the people who were clearly in my life just for the drinking or drug taking have, thankfully, disappeared. I have been quite brutal in distancing myself from anyone who was bad for my state of mind. People who made me feel shit about myself (maybe because they felt shit about themselves) or people who were always on the take and the make. They had to go. I realised you could forgive people but, at the same time, resolve to never really engage with them ever again.

Beyond my wife and two kids (plus my cat, Nelson, who has stuck by me even throughout the cocaine years when he would observe me mournfully while I chopped out lines on the kitchen surfaces at 3 a.m., shaking his head as if to say, 'You don't need to live like this, Dad'), I have built a wider squad of people who have become crucial to my sanity.

I have my personal trainer, Jordan. He is a former champion boxer who has, over the past six years, taught me about the cathartic beauty of punching things in interesting and ever-more elaborate combinations. Jordan isn't preachy but he does have the odd killer line up his sleeve. When I tell him I've been too busy with work to exercise he always says, 'Health before wealth, Sam.' But I get on with him. We talk about football and *The Sopranos* mostly. I look forward to seeing him every Thursday and Saturday morning (my son joins us for the Saturday training) – despite the fact that I almost always come away from our sessions feeling nauseous and faint.

Exercise gives me focus and energy. And being physically fit serves as a reminder of where I am and where I've come from. In the last couple of years of my drinking I had stopped exercising altogether and got really out of shape. Today, I am not exactly Chris Hemsworth (I am forty-seven, crisps remain my favourite food and I still have a pretty decent gut) but I can run continuously for miles without getting tired, I can lift heavy stuff and I can smash the shit out of a punchbag when I am feeling stressed. I'm doing OK. I'm much better than I was, which makes me feel happy.

I also have my therapist, Lizann, who I FaceTime with every Wednesday. We talk about all sorts. It's not just all the 'tell me about your mother' bullshit you see in films. Sometimes I will fall into telling her funny stories from when I was a kid just because I get a kick out of making her laugh. Other times I will moan to her about work so I don't have to bore my wife with it. And sometimes we will get into deeper shit about my addictions.

Sometimes I come away from a therapy session with a life-changing revelation fizzing through my mind and soul. Sometimes I come away just feeling 10 per cent more relaxed because I've let off steam about something trivial that was bothering me. Either way, I never regret a therapy session and I stick to my appointments religiously.

I also have an actual shrink. Dr Campbell is a psychiatrist and top addiction specialist up the Priory. I see him every few months so we can talk about the medication I am on to help keep my nut straight. He is wildly intelligent but warm and funny too. Mostly he asks me questions about my work – he seems fascinated by the stuff I do in the media. Occasionally I get to thinking, *What the fuck am I doing here? This isn't psychiatry!* And then – BAM! – Dr Campbell casually chucks out an observation or insight into my inner life that triggers a full-scale epiphany and I walk away from the appointment feeling like a giant weight has been lifted from my shoulders.

So those are the key members of the Sanity Squad I have built around myself over the past seven years. They are important to me living a good, stable and happy life and they are worth every penny. I know not everyone can afford this stuff but talking and exercise come free. Just find the right people to do it with, they don't have to be professionals. They just need to have love and understanding (and possibly some

235

weights or at least a set of resistance bands). If in doubt, start with your GP. They are more used to talking to people about their troubled mind than you might think. You don't have to be on the verge of a nervous breakdown to make an appointment and tell the doc you need a break.

Whatever your situation, just do it. Scheduling time devoted to looking after your body and brain is really important. It's more important than work or hobbies or socialising. None of those things matter more than you being happy, healthy and stable. I started to prioritise all of that shit above almost everything else in my life a few years ago and it worked.

Work is just the stuff you do in your spare time. Looking after yourself is your real full-time job. Just make sure you've got the right people around you to do it.

31

The Day I Threw Dinner at Dad

You might remember that in June 2017 there was a pretty dramatic general election, which was followed a few days later by the Grenfell Tower tragedy. I was covering both for my daily radio show. It was probably the busiest period of my life. My company was thriving in the background but I had way too much on and I felt myself fraying at the edges. I became emotionally invested in Grenfell, covering the story live from the scene in the immediate aftermath amidst all the tears and rage and despair. I was drawn into the situation on a deeper level partly because it took place in a part of west London that had been my home for several years. But also because my head was all over the place at the time anyway: I hadn't had a drink for two years but I was what you might call 'stark-raving sober'. Work had replaced booze and drugs as my destructive obsession; I was now using my career as a means of distraction from the deeper emotional issues I had previously suppressed by getting battered six nights a week.

It was in this context that I ruined Father's Day on Sunday 18 June by throwing a plate of liver and bacon all over my dad in the middle of a fancy West End restaurant.

I had rocked up to this celebratory event feeling tired and disgruntled. My dad doesn't like my siblings and me making a fuss of him on such occasions and tries to avoid our calls and invites. We had eventually convinced him to let us take him for dinner by booking the most expensive place we could think of. He had attended begrudgingly. He can be a bit weird, my old man.

At some point between the starters and main course he had taken issue with a throwaway comment I had made about politicians being corrupt.

It was one of the many things I say daily that I haven't really thought through. But he picked me up on it and wouldn't leave it alone. I asked him to stop, explaining that I had just been talking shit, but for some reason he wouldn't let up. He interrogated and probed and dissected and niggled incessantly. I'm not quite sure what his agenda was but he seemed intent on verbally crushing me. I was so tired and anxious and muddle-headed. It was fucking horrible.

As he berated me for my idiocy, two of my older brothers sat by and heckled, laughing at his tirade from the sidelines. They had been drinking and seemed to want to ramp the whole situation up for their entertainment. My older sister just looked uncomfortable and embarrassed. I had arrived in a state of mental and emotional exhaustion that was not my dad's or anyone else's fault. They wouldn't have known I was a man on the edge. I'd like to think that, if they had, my brothers might not have goaded my dad on to further attack me. But who knows? What happened next was not anyone's fault but my own.

I told my dad to fuck off, loudly enough for the other diners in the swishy eatery to turn around and stare.

I momentarily hesitated and considered apologising. But, before I could, my dad tipped me over the edge by smirking and calling me 'pathetic'.

At that exact moment the waiter arrived with his main course: a plate of liver and bacon, served on a bed of creamy mash, smothered in rich onion gravy. I looked at my dad's sneering face. I looked at the sumptuous plate of food. The temptation was just too great. Reader, I chucked it at him.

I grabbed a fistful of the overpriced offal and launched it from close range at my father – the mad, brownish-red concoction exploded all over his crisp white shirt. Bullseye. He gawped in astonishment. The waiter froze in amazement. My brothers stopped sniggering. The whole restaurant fell momentarily silent but for the awkward clink of cutlery on china. My sister looked like she was going to cry. I turned and strutted out of the joint, giving the maître d' a cocky 'See ya' on my way.

I got on my scooter and rode home in the evening heat, fighting back tears the whole way.

I had swaggered out of the restaurant like Jack the Biscuit. But I was totally distraught. Yes, my dad had been a dick. That, to be honest, was nothing new. But I loved him. And I knew he loved me. And I'd always thought that his occasionally dickish tendencies were born out of other stuff in his life that I just didn't know about or understand.

Whatever, I just felt absolutely ashamed and disgusted with myself. I really wanted to hug him and tell him I loved him, and I wanted him to say the same thing back to me.

I don't know if you've ever thrown a plate of liver and bacon at your dad but, take it from me, it doesn't make you feel great about yourself.

When I got home, I staggered into the front room, slumped down on the sofa and poured everything out to my wife. Not just the mad events from the restaurant but the exhaustion, confusion and anxiety that had been plaguing me for the past few weeks. I had hidden all of it because I was ashamed of it. From the outside looking in, my life might have looked great. I didn't want to be that bloke moaning about the 'pressure' of his dream job or the 'stress' of raising a family. I am still embarrassed to be writing this stuff now. I know there are people out there who have tougher lives than mine was then or is now. I also know that there are loads of you reading this who have difficult relationships with your dad.

My dad can be a bit rude sometimes. Most people in his life have just let him get away with it. But I struggle to. I have a lot of resentment about the past, which I am trying my best to process. I've inherited his tendency to charge enthusiastically into conflict with people. As a result, my dad and I argue sometimes.

Two of my biggest hang-ups dovetailed immaculately on that fateful Father's Day: the sense that my dad looked down on me; and a little-brother complex, which made me particularly sensitive to my siblings' inebriated hectoring. My dad having a pop at my intelligence in a fancy restaurant while my pissed-up brothers cheered him on from the sidelines was a perfect storm as far as my psyche was concerned.

Like I say, I had been sober for two years but that sobriety had lulled me into a false sense of security about myself. I thought my head was straight and that I had conquered my demons. Clearly, I had not. I had stopped imbibing alcohol and drugs, yes. But that was where my sobriety began and ended. The underlying issues that I had been trying to drink, smoke and snort away for the best part of four decades were still

240

lurking there, as strong and poisonous as ever – dictating my barmy responses to situations like the one in that restaurant.

I've just read this back and noticed that I have referred to all of my feelings in the past tense as if they don't exist any more. That's bollocks – I still carry all of that shit with me. Resentment, shame, anger, insecurity and all the other crap. But since I slowed my life down a bit and addressed my sobriety more seriously, I have made a huge amount of progress. I notice when my insecurities are trying to make me act in unhelpful or stupid ways. I can reflect more calmly on stuff and prevent myself from flying off the handle. I have managed to get all those bad feelings under better control, so I don't walk around on an emotional knife edge all the time, one snide remark away from throwing food at someone.

My dad sent me a text later that evening, presumably after going home and changing his shirt.

He told me he was sorry for winding me up. I couldn't believe it. Apologies are not really his thing usually. I told him that I was sorry too. However much he had wound me up, my response had been wildly disproportionate. He was just being a grumpy old man. Whereas I was a strung-out lunatic.

The next day, I spoke about the incident in detail on my radio show for the best part of three hours. At the time, it felt like the most sensible way of processing things. Christ, no wonder the station didn't renew my contract.

When we were teens, my mates and I would spend almost all of our time physically together but emotionally apart. We were cruel to each other, to be honest. We found it funny and, most of the time, it was. We'd say mean shit, we'd fight, we'd attempt to sabotage each other – particularly when it came to girls. When you're a teenager, anxious about the state of your own love life, it can be painful to see your pals succeed romantically. So you'd try to trip each other up. Once, my mates set me up on a date with a girl they knew to be completely disinterested in me, as a prank. On whom? Both of us, I guess. They arranged to meet me at the cinema but never turned up. Instead, this girl turned up alone – having assumed, like me, it was a group outing. She was extremely uncomfortable and so was I. They had told her, it transpired, that I was slightly obsessed with her. She assumed I'd masterminded the whole set up. As it happened, I wasn't in the least bit interested in her anyway. (Yeah, I know, I still sound like a sulky teen who is protesting too much over the matter but I am telling you, I DIDN'T EVEN FANCY HER, OK!) Anyway, we agreed not to watch the movie together and went our separate ways. But the rumour was now out there that I had contrived a date with this girl, which made me look like a bit of a weirdo.

My best mates were all still around when I decided to get sober. The ones who had helped me (unwittingly) forge the foundations of my drink and drug problems in the first place. A handful of lads I met at school (a couple of them at nursery) and hadn't shaken off since. They were, like me, complete wankers. But they were my wankers. I didn't want to live without them.

We'd drunk, popped, snorted and laughed our tits off with each other non-stop since the last days of Thatcher right through to the ghastly reign of David 'Shitface' Cameron. Beers and bongs in the park when we were barely shaving. Fingering girls in the sand bunker at the crazy golf. Holidays in the Costa Brava, smashed off our tits and locked out of the campsite at 3 a.m. Coke in West End khazis. Pills and carnivals. Deaths, marriages, births and divorces. We had been through it all together. But was there anything of any real substance there, behind all the hedonism and piss-taking?

When I decided to stop drinking, I didn't know what to expect from them.

One by one, I let my old mates know about my decision. They knew me well enough to know I was serious. Their response was so beautiful. There was no fanfare or inquest. No judgements or piss-taking. They were unflinching. All of them simply got on with our friendship. They bought me lemonades or made me cups of tea and never bothered me with tedious cross-examinations.

They pretty much acted like they didn't give a fuck – which is exactly what I needed. When you first quit drink, you don't want it to be a big deal that you must keep discussing. You're still straightening your own head out. You don't have any answers yet. My mates gave me space and time to work it out. Slowly, after some years, I started to open up here and there. They knew what I needed. It was a case of caring by not oversharing.

They never left me out of plans or complained about me being boring (to be fair, I am never boring). They never did that thing of drunkenly imploring me to have 'just the one for old times' sake'. These men had bigger hearts and more sensitivity than I could have ever imagined.

What they did for me was so quietly powerful.

I didn't want to lose my entire identity just because I wasn't drinking. I didn't want to hand in my Jack the Lad card. They let me keep it. They showed me that I was still the same old Sam – noisy, funny, full of shit – only sober. And that was enough for them.

Recovery has made me more open and reflective with everyone I know. I've seen my mates slowly start to move in the same direction as they get older.

On the sly, when no one else is listening, each of them has told me they are proud of me. What they don't realise is the massive part they played in my sobriety. The deeper meaning of my friendships has been one of best discoveries of sober life. There were times in the past when I might have thought my mates were just dickheads I got drunk with. It turned out that they were my brothers – beautiful humans with gigantic hearts and incredible sensitivity that had been hidden for so long beneath all the beer and banter.

It is there in everyone.

32

Therapy Is Much More of a Laugh Than You Think

The first time I went to see a therapist I was shitting myself. Not just about what he might ask me ('No mate, I do not fancy my mum') but mainly about anyone else finding out.

I had this furtive phone call with a bloke over the phone who gave me his address – a mews house in a fancy part of town. On my way, I was really worried that I might bump into someone I knew and blurt out what I was up to.

Guess what? I really did bump into someone I knew. I was at Earl's Court station when a bloke I knew from West Ham approached and asked, as people do when they encounter each other at a train station, where I was off to.

I doubt he really cared where I was off to. It was just something to say. But I panicked and started babbling on about a totally fictitious work meeting.

Back then, telling him that I was off to see a therapist felt akin to telling him I was going to a sex dungeon to have my bollocks electrocuted by an old man dressed as a gimp. In fact, at least that would have made me seem a bit adventurous and colourful. But therapy? Paying someone to listen to me whinge about my perfectly normal life? It was an unthinkable admission.

The importance of sharing has become a bit of a wanky cliché but it is 100 per cent legit. Sharing is essential to keeping your nut straight. There are a million reasons why but here are some of the key ones:

1. By sharing your feelings you discover that other people feel the same way – you are not weird and don't need to feel ashamed. Getting depressed or anxious is as normal as getting a cold in December. And it doesn't make you weak either – Churchill was always getting depressed and that nutter beat Hitler.

2. Sometimes our feelings are the result of an overloaded mind. The culture we live in is way too frantic and overflowing with demented stimuli. Your brain ends up looking like the drawer you keep all your headphones and charger cables in: a tangled-up mess. To untangle it you need to start addressing your worries and problems one by one. Saying them out loud to a sympathetic and non-judgemental listener makes it a thousand times easier.

3. Recognising your pain. Yes, that sounds a bit wanky too. 'What pain?' you might ask. We all live in the land of milk and honey – with flushing toilets, iPads and a Deliveroo attending to our every whim. We have nothing to complain about. Well, yes. But that's all material comfort. It doesn't protect you from emotional pain. All of us have had bits

and bobs of that stuff our whole lives. And most people – men in particular – become adept at hiding that pain from themselves and others because we're conditioned to 'suck it up' and 'just get on with it'. As a result, all the little cuts and bruises start to accumulate into bigger scars. And they can keep getting bigger until you acknowledge and then address them. Therapy helps you do this. You can look at your life honestly and identify the stuff that might have had a negative effect on you along the way. You might even sympathise with yourself a bit. Which, in turn, will at least make you stop feeling so guilty about feeling shit.

Therapy is great for all of the above and so much more. It makes your head and your heart fitter and stronger, allowing you to manage your life better and face down the inevitable challenges you encounter along the way.

Some popular myths about therapy are that it's for hippies sitting about on beanbags and getting you to scream at the memory of a kid who bullied you at school (maybe this type of therapy exists – probably in the Brighton area – but it is rare and easily avoided). Or that it involves some German-sounding shrink in a pair of half-moon specs trying to convince you that your parents were both cunts.

The truth is that there are all sorts of therapists out there and few of them conform to the daft clichés. You are likely to meet someone smart, compassionate, non-judgemental and well trained in helping you combat the stuff that is making you feel shit.

Yes, you might have to shop around until you find someone with whom you click. But when you do (and you will), you will find that talking to someone who has no emotional investment in your problems is incredibly liberating. You open up about your feelings to an extent you never previously thought possible. And the more you do so, the more they can help you.

I prefer getting stuff off my chest to a paid pro during my weekly Wednesday session than making my wife have to listen to it non stop.

If you can't afford a therapist or are having to wait for a referral please talk to a friend or relative about your troubles. There are always people who will listen. Your problems are never as big as they seem. They just need a bit of untangling. Use the helpful contact details at the back of the book if you need someone to talk to right now.

And if, like me, you've already gone through the looking glass and found comfort in therapy, remember to be noisy about it. Let's normalise talking about this shit. Let's make going to a therapist as unremarkable as going to the dental hygienist.

Come on, lads, it's 2022 for fuck's sake. You don't have to pretend to be Clint Eastwood any more.

33

Sitting with Your Pain

Sometimes you can just have a little run of feeling down in the dumps for no apparent reason at all. My dad told me when I was younger that this was simply a 'hormonal matter' that needed to be waited out. There is some truth in that, I guess.

But sometimes you genuinely have a streak of bad luck. You experience an accumulation of very real, perfectly tangible problems all at once and it leaves you feeling legitimately miserable.

It was winter 2021 and I was having a run of bad luck. I won't bore you with all of the details but, in summary, they involved my wife having to go into hospital for a while (nothing serious), a really bad back, an unexpected financial blow, a recent tooth removal that left my mouth in significant pain and a really fucking bad sore throat, which landed me in bed for most of the week.

Poor me. Isn't my life hard? Well, yes and no. On the one hand, all of the little inconveniences listed above were genuine sources of stress and the accumulation of them all was a pain in the arse (as well as the back, mouth and throat). OK, I didn't have cancer. But so what? The bar doesn't have to be set that high, does it? Problems are problems even when they're not life threatening.

It is natural to have problems. It is unlucky for them all to come at once, yes, but that happens to all of us from time to time.

I am warming to the idea that mild suffering is our natural state. I find the idea quite comforting. In the past, when I was constantly trying to swim against the tide of melancholy, I found it hard to accept bad times.

But back in winter 2021 I noticed something strange happening. I didn't feel anxious or depressed. I didn't even feel particularly sorry for myself. I did not waste time speculating about worst-case scenarios. I did not start reading deep, dark things into the bad luck that had beset me. I just felt a bit miserable. But feeling a bit miserable is normal. I felt quite good about feeling miserable, to be honest.

The writer and philosopher Alain de Botton calls this a state of 'sane insanity'; a grasp of our own imperfections and an acceptance of life's natural frustrations. When faced with problems, the sanely insane don't get angry, bitter or resentful. They don't feel as if they have been singled out by a vindictive universe. They realise that this sort of stuff is as much a part of the human experience as breathing air. They accept the pain and recognise their own torment. As American bumper stickers put it: shit happens.

For years I suffered from the delusion that a perfect, problem-free life was possible. We live in a world that aggressively promotes the idea that an ideal life, defined by non-stop success, buoyancy and LOLs, actually exists. We see signs every day, on our phones, on our TV sets, plastered all over the side of buses

– that other people are actually living these lives. And so, when we are suffering, we feel doubly bad because it's like we're the only ones. That everyone else is at a fantastic party while we are stuck at home cleaning out the U-bend of the toilet. *Why am I having such a shitty time?* we wonder. *Maybe because I am weak or stupid or cursed!* These thoughts can make us feel ashamed. We deny our problems to ourselves and others. The problems seem bigger, we feel even more isolated and so the whole shit-show goes on and on.

When times are tough try to remember the following:

1. Of course times are tough. That's life. Good times are the exception, bad times are the rule. Don't read anything into it beyond the fact that you are human and this is all part of the experience.

2. Of course you feel miserable about the problems you're facing. Who wouldn't? Feeling sad about sad things is not a sign of weakness or insanity. It is just a normal response to shit things happening. Accept it and embrace it. Your situation might still be shit but acknowledging it as such will help you deal with it better.

3. Everyone feels the same as you. We might live in a society that discourages people from sharing stuff about how shit they feel. But they do feel shit. Not always, but a great deal of the time. You are not alone in this. You are not weak for feeling this way. It is totes normal.

4. Tell people how you feel. Hiding it makes it worse for you. And sharing it will help others who are suffering in the same way. Pass this shit on.

So that's it. Like anyone, problems pass through my life from time to time. Like anyone, I sometimes whinge about them. But, finally, I think I've got my troubles in some sort of perspective. I have started to react to bad times in a more appropriate way: not with panic or rage but with a reasonable level of sadness and annoyance. Rather than see my life as a corny movie, and this little period as the tragic final act, I am finally able to realise that this is all just a journey. I am watching my problems float past me like empty cans of Tennent's on the canal. They'll be gone soon. Then I can look up at the sky, smell the trees, have a snack and enjoy life's little pleasures for a bit. Until the next set comes along.

34

How Not to Listen

Opening up is great. I've made my feelings on that abundantly clear. But in order for it to work, we need other people to listen to us. Sometimes we might be the ones who need to listen to someone else. There is an art to listening, although it's one I have yet to master. I'd actually go as far as to say that – sometimes – I am shit at listening.

Often what people need is an understanding, sympathetic and non-judgemental audience. Someone who can sit there and consume what is being said with focus. Nodding often helps. A small smile where appropriate. A little frown occasionally to demonstrate empathy. Maybe even an arm round the shoulder. Certainly, these are the things I appreciate when I'm opening up to someone.

But when I'm on the other end of things I struggle to just keep my ears open and my big mouth shut. I have a tendency to offer advice. Or tell the other person how the thing they are going through is really similar to a thing I myself have been through in the past. Sometimes I just try to gee up the other person with a pseudo-Churchillian call to arms.

Why do I feel the need to do this? Why can't I just shut up and listen? Maybe it's ego. I want to demonstrate to the other person that I am wise and experienced and have a solution to all of their problems. As if they have simply told me they have a headache and I am explaining to them the benefits of Ibuprofen.

It's also because I am so desperate to show the other person that I care, I understand and that I have been through similar shit myself – so they needn't feel awkward about opening up to me. I babble excitedly about my own experiences as if to say: *It's OK. You are safe here. I too am riddled with inner turmoil! We are in the same gang!*

But I don't think any of this is particularly helpful. I guess it's just pathological. But I am working on it.

Aside from all of that, I just talk out of awkwardness. I simply hate long silences. I feel like if I listen to their problems and then don't say something meaningful in response I will come across as disinterested. So, like a dickhead with a Jesus complex, I set about trying to talk someone out of ever being sad again.

And the thing is, I always come away from those conversations feeling a bit shit about myself. Because all I want to do is be there for people I care about and show them a sympathetic ear. But too often it feels like I am making the conversation all about me.

There is no punchline or learning to any of this. I am not about to tell you how I have learned to be a better listener. I have not. I remain a shit listener. But at least I now understand that I am a shit listener and I'm trying to do something about it. Someone sent me an affirmation this week that was titled 'Please, Just Listen'. (I don't think the person who sent this was aiming it at me personally, but who knows?)

Here is a bit from it that resonated with me and I will try to bear in mind . . .

'I don't need advice. I do need you to reflect my feelings by listening then helping me to see my own choices. Then I will listen to you.'

35

How to Be (Quite) Happy

My son Lenny, who is ten, started his own podcast. It's all about an imaginary football universe he started creating a few years ago. It was so vast, detailed, mad and hilarious that I began mentioning it on my own podcast, *Top Flight Time Machine*. Listeners seemed to like it.

So now Len has started his own thing and asked me to be co-host and producer. He is very serious about it, writing proper running orders and topic outlines before we record. He is even learning to edit it himself. In a way, I hope he doesn't learn how to do it all himself too quickly because then I might be redundant. For the time being, working on the podcast with him is enormously fulfilling for me. He's learning some useful creative skills, yes, but more than that, it's just a fun way for us to spend time together.

I'm telling you about this because I am proud of my son. But also because I want to focus a bit more on the little sources of joy that can make life so beautiful. I've written a great deal in this book about dark times and struggles and how to overcome adversity. I have done so in order to show other people that they are not alone in sometimes feeling overwhelmed, scared, worried, frustrated or ashamed.

But, you know, life isn't all shit. Loads of it is wonderful. The trick is to spot the wonderful bits as they happen and really savour them.

That said, no one likes a smug cunt. There are plenty of people who write about mental health while simultaneously boasting about their own incredibly successful and serene existences. Which, ultimately, only contributes to the feelings of inadequacy that many of their readers are trying to overcome.

So I usually swerve writing too much about the good times.

But I will tell you this. My daughter, Coco, is fifteen and easily the funniest person I know. She holds court at our dining table twice every day – at breakfast and dinner. She is not one of those loud, annoying teenagers. Her humour is gently acerbic; it feels like being slapped in the face with a velvet glove. She batters and bemuses me with her words. Sometimes she manages it with just a roll of her eyes. She belittles and condemns me in a way that only your own offspring really can. She cuts right to my very core with a smile and a wink and I love her for it.

She keeps my feet on the ground and often makes me confront the daft truth about myself. But the way in which she does it, with so much eloquence and wit, just makes me swell with pride. I've always considered myself an elite-level piss-taker and have dished out loads to my own parents over the years. But Coco does it at a level I could never dream of. Her banter is psychedelic. But all of it is infused with love. Sometimes the two of us just go out for a drive so we can chat shit to each other for an hour or so without bothering anyone else. Time with her is a privilege.

This pair, together with Anna who is the love of my life, are the centre of my universe.

My life is pretty simple and small these days. I spend a great deal of it sitting round a table with these three legends, sharing jokes and stories from our days. Showing interest in each other, taking the piss, mucking about, talking shit and losing ourselves in the beauty of it all. These are the moments I try to celebrate inside. I'm sorry if it makes me smug. But I am telling you all of this as a reminder to celebrate your own little moments of joy, whatever they might be.

I spent a great deal of my younger life expecting fulfilment and euphoria to be delivered by massive, extravagant moments: money, success, fame, status, the respect of strangers, blow jobs and charlie and first-class flights and three-nil victories under the floodlights.

But it's all a big red herring. The joy in life is all around us all the time and often simpler than we have been conditioned to expect. It's all about where you put your focus. These days, mine is trained solely on that dining table and the people who share it with me. Plus the cat, of course. Fuck me, if I didn't have Nelson to talk to when I was feeling low I don't know what I'd do. Whoever you are, you should really think about getting a cat.

Nelson is almost fourteen in human years. He has had a tough life. I bought him off a woman outside Hammersmith station for seventy quid. The vet told me he was too young to have been taken from his mum and would probably die. But he didn't; we diligently nursed him through his early days and, I think, a special bond was formed between us as a result.

In our first house, he was bullied by the neighbours' cats: a couple of unscrupulous Russian blues called Oscar and Archie. They used to chase Nelson around the garden and even into our house. He was in a constant state of fear, which he expressed by 'over-grooming' his belly until it went bald. The vet prescribed cat-Valium, which we had to crush up in his food. They also flogged me a plug-in pheromone diffuser supposedly designed to relax cats. It cost me about fifty quid. My mum called me a 'stupid cunt' for buying that. Whatever, Mum.

When we moved house, Nelson had to move in with my mother-in-law for a few months because the builders were renovating the new place. While there, Nelson was bullied once again by a local tabby called Bunny. Bunny was a prick and his owners did little to control his antisocial behaviour. Nelson started over-grooming again.

At the start of lockdown, Nelson got his tail slammed in the back door (a gust of sudden wind blew it shut on him). He was smashed to fuck and had to have two operations. We thought it was going to be amputated at one point. He's better now.

Despite all of his struggles, Nelson seems happy today. He is sitting beside me right now, like he always is when I am writing. When I finish work and sit on the sofa, he climbs up on my chest and claws gently at me, purring intensely right into my face. It's a bit full-on but eventually he settles down, stops clawing and just allows me to gently stroke his head while I watch telly. He means a great deal to me. Having him with me can be a genuine help when I am feeling tense or anxious. The love he shows me, the therapeutic sound of his purr and the soft, soothing touch of his fur.

I love the bastard. But I wouldn't want to be him. People are always on about cats having a nice easy life. But Nelson is a nervous wreck. I've got the vet's bills to prove it. Maybe I should buy him his own cat.

36

Glamorise Rest

They say that if you want something done, ask a busy person. That's true, if you don't mind it being done shit.

I have a track record of making shit decisions when I am over busy. Here's a couple of reasons why:

1. When I am over busy I get tired. And when I am tired my brain doesn't function properly – I become preoccupied with just getting things done as opposed to getting them right. So I make quickfire decisions just to get shit out of the way.

2. Conversely, being busy can make me overly confident in myself. If I am really busy I figure it must mean I am doing something right; that I am very good at my job, which is why so many people want to work with me. And so I breezily fire off ill-thought-through decisions in a sort of semi-psychotic state of hubris. I put an immense amount of faith in my natural instincts. But my natural instincts often suck. My rational brain is much more of a reliable influence.

But it's really hard to be rational when you are strung out and knackered.

Being busy is overrated. It is also counter-productive: you think you're getting stuff done by filling every moment of your day but, with no time to breathe or reflect on any of your decisions, you end up doing everything half-arsed.

The government are always telling us how many pieces of fruit and veg we should eat or how many units of alcohol we should drink. Why don't they shout as loudly about the amount of hours we should be working? Young people joining the workforce just don't know this stuff. No one warns them about overwork. In fact, they do the opposite: kids are told that the way to get on is to keep your head down, your mouth shut and your eyes off the clock. Only by devoting yourself completely to 'the grind' will you get the attention of the bosses and the progression you desire. Well, I've been on both sides of that lie so I know exactly what a scam it is.

Thatcher's been dead for around a decade and yet so many of us still buy into the bullshit she sold us about hard work being its own reward. Like fuck it is. Hard work is a conspiracy; a scam conjured up by the bosses to enslave us all and give us bad backs. Our worth is not intrinsically linked to our productivity.

I'm not some sort of fucking hippy. I don't think we all need to start living in communes and having it off with each other's wives. And I'm not a communist either. I think work is necessary and can be liberating too. Sometimes, it can even be enjoyable. It's the grind that's the problem. Working your arse off for insufficient rewards, neglecting your mental and physical health, numbing the sense of exhaustion with booze, drugs and shitty food – and all the while bragging about it.

I spent so long being the sort of prick who prided himself on how busy he was. 'How are you?' people would ask. 'Good,' I'd say. 'Busy.' As if the two things went hand in hand. Then I would roll my eyes as if to say: *What am I gonna do? I can't help being in demand and extraordinary. Luckily I can cope with the crazy schedule because I am such a fucking legend.* I was not a fucking legend. I was a fucking twat.

I got addicted to being busy for the same reason I got addicted to booze and drugs. I was scared. Scared of slowing down and just seeing what happened. Scared of what fresh horrors life might have waiting for me around every corner. Just scared of being alive. Work was a brilliant distraction from all that stuff. And unlike getting constantly pissed or high, work addiction attracted praise and admiration from people. But it shouldn't have done.

People should stop fetishising work. They should stop glorifying grafters. They should stop glamorising the grind. The grind is bollocks. Not only does it make you miserable, knackered and unhealthy – it also makes you shit at your job. We should start glamorising rest instead.

Businesses are obsessed with constantly increasing profits. The economy is in flux. And so everyone asks their workers to do more for less. It's the quickest and easiest way to protect margins. They incentivise workers by promising career progression and increased opportunities. But we all know that's bullshit. We work hard because we don't want to lose our jobs and starve to death. It's pretty ugly if you stop to think about it in such stark terms – which is why we just keep working to distract ourselves instead.

I appreciate that I claimed earlier that I wasn't a communist and yet here I am, just five paragraphs later, sounding very much like a fucking communist. But I love capitalism. I like money and enjoy buying stuff. I think that ambition is normal and the market can be an engine of progress. I just think modern capitalism is getting a bit silly and unimaginative. There must be a better way of moving the world forward than just working everyone harder and harder and harder. What did we invent robots and Zoom calls for? I'm all for profit. But there are smarter ways to pursue it than grinding everyone into physical and emotional wrecks. And by the way, I also understand that jobs are essential for survival and it's easy for me to sit here knocking this bollocks out on an Apple Mac when I don't have to work three shifts a day just to cover the rent.

But whatever you do – whether you're a cleaner or a CEO – you still need to rest and you shouldn't be expected to work at the pace of a machine just to survive. We might not be able to smash the system overnight but we can at least try to go a bit easier on ourselves, whatever we do for a living.

As I've said, when I was a kid my mum worked as a secretary in offices she often hated. Then she became a carer for old people, which was slightly more fulfilling but much harder and more poorly paid. To me she was a hero – working all hours to support her four sons. So whenever I felt that my relatively easy life of writing books and being on telly was getting too much for me, I told myself that I had no right to feel tired. But we all have the right to feel tired and to do something about it.

It is so obvious to me now that overwork was one of the biggest factors in my boozing and drug taking in my twenties and thirties. I was self-employed and would never say no to more work, however overstretched I was. Anxiety and constant insecurity haunted me even when I was earning well. I assumed every job would be my last. When I had kids I thought I would calm down but the added sense of responsibility only made me worse. I never rested – I just punctuated the work with getting battered. I had to anaesthetise myself from the pressures of the grind. What kind of life requires constant artificial stimulants to make it manageable? That's fucking mental.

Let's glamorise rest. Let's make putting our feet up sexy. Let's focus less on our productivity and more on our leisurewear choices.

Resting is a cure all. Switching off your mind and your body can fix all of your problems: mental, emotional and physical. And I don't just mean weird stuff like yoga and complicated breathing techniques. I mean watching a film and having a bag of Quavers on the sofa. Have a nap. Or go for a run. Just do shit you like. Mindless stuff. Put time aside for it. Treat yourself to it. Take pride in the amount of time you spend doing fuck all. Learn to pity the dickheads who boast about how busy they are. They are insecure, scared and miserable. Try to help them if you can.

The grind is bullshit. Your sofa is your friend. We all need money, yes. But quit giving more than you're being paid for on the empty promise that it will one day bring you riches. It probably won't. Quit thinking that staying late at the office makes you look tough or cool or dynamic. It definitely doesn't.

Be a shirker, not a worker.

37

How to Help an Addict

'You think I'm bad person.'

That was the message my mate sent me when I had floated the idea that he might be a drug addict.

That's what he wanted to believe. He was trapped in a narcotic hellscape so warped that he thought the world was against him. It suited him to feel that way. He was thriving off anger and resentment. Those feelings were giving him the excuse he needed to keep using.

I knew all of this because it was how I felt for a long time before I got sober.

The only thing that helped me snap out of my bad behaviour was love. Criticism only fuelled my false sense of victimhood, which, in turn, drove me deeper into my addictions. It was only when people showed me love and understanding that I started to feel as if life might be worth living without drugs and alcohol.

Of course, it's really hard to remain patient and understanding when you have an addict in your life. It is perfectly fair if sometimes, when you have tried repeatedly to help them and they have persistently let you down, you just walk away. Sometimes you must to protect yourself.

But if you can manage it, always choose to show the addict that they are loved; that you can see they are going through something painful; that you might not understand exactly what that pain is, but you acknowledge it exists. That you realise they are not using drugs or booze just because they are weak or indulgent but that their life has got a bit too much for them and they could do with some help.

People can slip into addiction when life just gets too overwhelming. Often, it's because they haven't dealt with bad feelings from the past. Or maybe the stresses and strains of the here and now are just starting to suffocate them. They don't feel like they can talk about any of the stuff that is making them feel shit because they think it will make them sound weak, pathetic or self-indulgent. And so they leave all the pain inside where it ferments, getting stronger every day. Drugs or alcohol provide the easiest way out.

If you shout at them, tell them they are being selfish or weak or pathetic, then you are confirming all of their worst fears. They will dive deeper into their addictions. But if you tell them that you love them, you believe in them and it's OK for them to admit to feeling shit, then you have a much better chance of getting through to them. You might not fix their addiction overnight. But you might just plant a seed in their head that tells them that the world isn't quite such a harsh and judgemental place. That they are not such a shitty person. And that a different life, free from the control of their addictions, might be possible.

It's not easy to show an addict love and understanding because addicts often act like arseholes. Don't feel bad about yourself if you are just too exhausted and exasperated by their antics to show love and understanding. You are not obliged to fix them.

I'm just saying that, if you feel inclined to help, then love is the key.

'I don't think you're a bad person, I think you're a beautiful person and I love you,' I replied to my mate.

A bit weird, sure. But it got him to sit up and listen, I reckon.

38

How to Ignore Your Own Thoughts

It was my son's tenth birthday party. We had a few of his mates round to go mental and fuck about in the superb way that only ten-year-old boys can. I stood back from the action, realising that they had now reached an age where they no longer found my banter and antics ('bantics') amusing.

I was happy to just loiter in the kitchen, monitoring the snacks. There were so many snacks. The sort of snacks that, ordinarily, my wife goes to great lengths to hide from me. She knows what I am like. I am an addict. I might have managed to stay off the booze and gear for the past few years but I am prone to channel my batshit appetites and manic compulsions into whatever else is put in front of me.

At the birthday party, I was left unguarded around the pickled onion Monster Munch. And so I ate them. Sacks and sacks of them. I was more Monster Munch than man by the end of the party. After nibbling just one, something was triggered inside my brain. Nostalgic recall of childhood comfort eating perhaps, like Proust with his madeleines. Delaney and his pickled onion

Monster Munch. My dopamine system was activated. The happy hormones pulsed through my body and that was it, I was gorging on them like a fat sultan for the rest of the afternoon. Onlookers noted that my eyes glassed over as if the tartly flavoured snacks had sent me into a kind of trance. Lovely.

The consequences of this binge were mildly unpleasant. I felt sick and emotionally fragile for the rest of the day. I was dehydrated and unsettled. Self-hatred set in around the time that the other parents began knocking at the door to pick up their kids. I saw some of them glance furtively at the tell-tale crumbs on my face and jumper. I felt judged. I was ashamed. And so I ate more. Fucking hell.

My brain has always been obsessive. It latches on to one thought and won't let go of it until I am almost broken. Saturday's thought was 'MUST EAT MONSTER MUNCH'. Someone with a more disciplined mind would probably enjoy just a handful of Monster Munch and think to themselves: *What a mildly pleasing interlude in my day this has been. Now it's time to get on with the rest of my life.* Whereas I think: *Jesus Christ! Monster Munch are delicious! Eating them is all I ever want to do for the rest of my life! FUCK SOCIETY! SMASH THE SYSTEM!*

And I won't stop until I am sick or crying, or my wife stages an intervention.

Booze, drugs, shopping, spending, Monster Munch. It's all the fucking same. When I experience pleasure I just want more. Equally, my brain can attach itself limpet-like to negative feelings like fear or shame or worry. The overarching problem is an inability to break a certain line of thought. Once a notion has its hooks in my brain, I can struggle to think about anything else.

I'm an obsessive thinker. Like many other people, my brain has the capacity to operate on a loop system. But I've come to realise that I do have some control over it. I can manage my thought process rather than just accept (perhaps excuse) my obsessive tendencies as part of my genetic make-up. Which is a massive relief because, for large parts of my life, I have had to wrestle daily with barmy, destructive overthinking, which I always tried my best to hide behind a happy-go-lucky persona. I mean, no one wants to be thought of as a nervous ninny, do they?

A small worry can take hold and consume me for days on end.

Sometimes my ability to fixate so deeply on a particular thought has helped me complete projects or come up with great ideas. I am occasionally able to use my obsessive attitudes to help me get in physical shape or solve a big problem. I can be dogged and that can sometimes be useful. I will give up sugar completely for six months or stay up eight nights running to finish writing a book. But it's still not healthy and it can be fucking annoying for the people around me.

Worry, pleasure, fear, excitement: it doesn't matter if the thoughts drive feelings that are good or bad, the relentless cycle is the problem. The inability to just compartmentalise a particular thought and manage life in a balanced way – that seems to be at the heart of so many people's problems.

Who knows why some of us have more obsessive minds than others? Maybe we were so afraid or anxious in our childhoods that our brains just got moulded that way. Or maybe we were too indulged and just never learned when to stop. Maybe it's all innate and our brains are just wired to operate like broken record players. Mind you, I once interviewed a brain surgeon who explained that, while it's true that we can develop physical patterns in the brain that drive obsessive thoughts, it is also possible to reshape those patterns. Just like lifting weights can change the shape of our limbs, being focused in our thinking can change the shape of our brains. That's what he says anyway.

I know that cognitive behavioural therapy has done wonders for loads of people. I've done a bit of that – although appealing to your brain's more rational impulses sometimes feels a bit ambitious when you are riddled with deeply emotional, wildly confusing thoughts that you know are mental but you just can't stop.

What I do nowadays is just ignore my thoughts more often. I used to take my own brain way too seriously. If the seed of something negative drifted through my mind I would jump on it and nurture it into a gigantic shitstorm. Equally, I would identify some small source of pleasure such as food or drugs or drink or even just making someone laugh – and I would not stop milking it again and again and again until it stopped being fun.

It's hard to dig yourself out of these compulsive states once you are balls deep in them. So instead, I try to stave them off before they get a chance to take hold. I observe my thoughts more consciously. I see the potentially bad shit that might flutter into my brain throughout the day, and I quickly tell it to 'fuck off' before it gets too comfortable. If someone has annoyed me, I will spot a resentful response brewing in my mind and try to shut it down right away. I will simply think about something else until the moment has passed. I will actively try to change the subject in my mind. I will sit back and just wait for the thought to go away. I remind myself that just because the thought exists, it doesn't necessarily deserve my attention or respect.

I trust my brain a lot less than I used to. I am vigilant. I try to better police my thoughts. I try to organise them into appropriate mental folders. Legitimate worries are set aside for a bit of rational reflection at an appropriate time. Indulgent compulsions are identified and disciplined robustly. Proper mad shit is dragged directly to trash. It has taken me forty-seven years but I feel like I am finally starting to take control of my own brain.

39

The Beauty of Letting Go

My laptop shut itself down one day and just never woke up again. It was dead. There was no warning. It was still quite young: eighteen months! That's no age. They couldn't work it out at the Apple Store. 'Sometimes, these things just happen,' the well-spoken nerd at the Genius Bar told me, his hand softly touching my shoulder in consolation.

I took it over to John Lewis. Those are the bastards that originally sold it to me. They said they would send it off to their 'menders'. I told them it was pointless but they insisted it was company policy. I waited patiently for three weeks, trying to get my work done on an iPad and my phone.

When it came back from the menders they said it was mended. But they lied. I took it home, switched it on, it blinked to life and said hello. Then, midway through recording a podcast about West Ham's defeat to Wolverhampton Wanderers, it died all over again. Imagine that! Having to go through the trauma and grieving process twice!

My entire life revolved around that laptop. I wrote stuff

and recorded stuff on to it for a living. It was what kept a roof over our heads. Everything was lost. My life ground to a halt without that laptop.

But, you know, fuck it. There is always a work around. I borrowed my daughter's laptop. I can pick up emails anywhere. If someone needed to contact me they found a way.

These thoughts might seem obvious to you but they represent a massive mental breakthrough for me. In the past, I would have shouted and screamed about something like that. I would have raised hell at the Apple Store and unleashed mayhem at John Lewis customer service. I would have ranted and raved until someone made it better. And while I behaved in this manner, those around me like my wife and kids would have had to watch on, accept my insanity and just quietly think to themselves, *What a silly bastard.*

It has taken me years to realise that I can't control the things that happen around me, only my reaction to those things. Going crazy, getting angry, seeking retribution or my own entitled sense of justice served little purpose other than raising my blood pressure.

It's no one's fault that my laptop broke. John Lewis tried their best to fix it, I'm sure. It was just something that happened, and I told myself that a resolution would eventually be found. Which it was – they eventually got it fixed and it all ended happily.

I was so proud of myself for practising a bit of patience. Traditionally, I am impatient and self-indulgent. It can hurt people around me. But the person it hurts most of all is me.

I have been working on fixing this shit in my head for a while now. But you never know if you're really fixed until a challenge comes along and tests you. The laptop breaking was a challenge. And here I am boasting to you about it. Boasting about my success in not behaving like a fucking toddler. Go me!

Well, we are all trying to become better in our own small ways. I'm seeking progress, not perfection. Acceptance, patience and a philosophical shrug of the shoulders in the face of minor inconvenience represents a giant stride forward for me. Like everyone else, I spend a great deal of time beating myself up for my flaws and failings. So once in a while, when I spot a tiny little bit of progress, I think it's OK to give myself a very, very small round of applause. You should make sure you do the same.

40

How to Be Wrong

I got a call from a broadcaster who wanted me to take part in a discussion about the war in Ukraine. That's right, me, Sam Delaney, the semi-anonymous podcaster, West Ham fan, former gossip magazine editor and suburban dad. They were going to pay me to express my opinions on the biggest geopolitical crisis of our times. It was the easiest fifty quid I've ever said no to.

The world is full of way too many opinions and the last thing I want to do is add mine to the disgusting mix (and, yes, I know that this book is full of my opinions – all of which I sincerely apologise for). Rolling news and social media mean that every gobshite in the world has the ability – and, even more worryingly, the inclination – to express their hot-take on everything. At times of genuine global crisis it can be a bit depressing. All these people trying to exploit human suffering to elevate their profile or further their career.

The fact that a legitimate outlet would want to fill airtime with the completely irrelevant viewpoint of someone like me is a shameful reflection of the level to which public discourse has sunk.

I should say that, in the past, I spent many years being a gobshite for hire on various TV and radio outlets doing just this sort of stuff. I was a whore, willing to comment upon almost any news story, anywhere and at any time. From the BBC's *Today* programme to Lorraine Kelly's morning sofa jamboree – and organs of various credibility in between – the sound of me offering my lukewarm takes on everything from politics to pets was an unwelcome background noise for several years.

But then I stopped. The reason was that the game changed. It used to be that I could say something daft or facetious or flippant about a news story and the producers seemed perfectly satisfied. It wasn't the earth-shattering, game-changing insight they were looking for. It was a bit of chatty relief from the more serious and boring business of actual news reporting. Real opinions were left to experts or at least brainier journalists than me.

Then, probably around the time of the Brexit campaign, things changed and all us pundits started needing to have big, controversial, argumentative positions on everything. Whimsical opinion was no longer enough. Counter-intuitive convictions and combative invective were the order of the day. I didn't have nearly enough of that stuff in my locker so I realised that I could either start to contrive passionate, militant and slightly barmy opinions or just stop insulting everyone's intelligence and gracefully withdraw from the arena of hate.

I chose the latter. Or perhaps people just stopped asking me on to their shows because I was just too wishy-washy. Probably a bit of both.

One thing I've noticed about the madder, more aggressive opinions you see online and on-air is that they are disproportionately expressed by men. The world seems filled with furious fellas determined to have their opinions heard and agreed with. There is an angry, spittle-mouthed need among so many older blokes to be right about stuff all the time. Where does that come from? Maybe it's because they got so used to their gender putting them on a pedestal for so long. And now they're struggling to come to terms with the fact that their perspective is subject to the same scrutiny and scepticism as anyone else's.

It must be fucking exhausting to give so much of a shit about how seriously you are taken.

Being OK with being wrong is so liberating. I sometimes get angry or frustrated in my personal life. Friends, family or colleagues might not appreciate my point of view or say something that upsets me. What I find helpful is to always reflect on arguments with the thought, *What was my part in that?* It doesn't mean that I always put myself in the wrong. It's just an acknowledgement of the fact that I can't control what other people say, do or think so it's pointless stewing on any of that. I can only control my own conduct. And anyway, there is absolutely always some way in which I really was wrong.

Bill Bernbach, the godfather of modern advertising, was said to have always carried a piece of paper in his pocket that read: 'Maybe he's right.'

Whatever happens, the best part of arguments is the bit where you get to say sorry afterwards. Once you've realised the part you played in a disagreement, it's great to go back to the other person and apologise. It never means you're taking all the blame. It just means you've got the intelligence to understand what really happened and the bollocks to admit it. That takes strength. I say sorry about half-a-dozen times a week these days. It's a great feeling, I can tell you.

Epilogue

Real Men Love Otters

I went up the local wetlands centre to see the otters on a Tuesday morning. The lads were on top form – splashing about in their otter lake, prancing about on their hindlegs, gobbling down bits of fish carcass like nobody's business. I love those little fellas. As always, the whole experience was truly life affirming.

I'd gone there with my mate Dan. He's just qualified as a personal trainer and is on a mission to help burned-out dads get their lives back on track. Like me, Dan has been sober for a few years now. Also like me, he knows what it's like to have charged headlong into fatherhood at 100 mph in his thirties only to crash a few years later, destroyed by work, stress and lack of sleep. Both of us, like so many other dads, turned to booze and drugs to try and cope. What a pair of dickheads.

Dan and I became mates from the football. We spent over a decade going to West Ham matches home and away, getting wankered, acting like pricks, watching our team lose in a variety of damp, freezing-cold locations. It was great.

Now those days are gone. It's not that we don't look back and treasure the memories. But we are more honest about the price we paid for those weekends of turbo-fuelled excess and mayhem. We always spent the days that followed in a state of regret and anguish; pain, shame and anxiety haunting our working week until the weekend came back around and we did it all over again.

It all gets a bit out of hand in the end.

Dan and I got sober around the same time. Giving up wasn't easy for either of us. But we got through it and now here we are on the other side – meeting up on a Tuesday morning to look at the otters. One thing we both reflected on, as we gazed upon the adorable semi-aquatic mammals, was how secretive we used to be about our own feelings.

Back then, I assumed I was the only one in our gang who worried and fretted for days after a binge. I thought I was the only one who woke up in the night consumed by guilt and self-hatred. I thought I was the only one frightened that I was deeply flawed and constantly teetering on the edge of failure. Turns out Dan was going through all those feelings too. For all I know, everyone we knew was. But in our twenties and thirties, no one wanted to show it.

In the pub on a Saturday, we were all so filled with the four Bs of the professional geezer: bravado, bullshit, booze and bugle. We were so eager to make each other laugh and just block out the shit that made us anxious during the week; we became experts at presenting ourselves as free-wheeling, carefree, laugh-a-minute legends. We all fooled each other into thinking that was our total reality.

Do I wish that we'd all been quieter and more reflective? That we'd sat around the pub drinking lemonade and talking about feelings? Do I fuck. Those days were great. But what

I've learned since then is that we can all have just as much of a laugh together without putting on a constant front. Getting sober, growing up and showing a bit of vulnerability doesn't mean you stop having fun.

Dan makes me laugh as much as he ever did. And – as you should have noticed by now, gentle reader – I remain fucking hilarious. But both of us are happy to admit the softer bits of our personalities; the feelings we've struggled with; the day-to-day shit that worries us; the residual insecurities we've carried around since we were kids. So what? I don't give a fuck if people know I'm flawed, insecure and half barmy. Being sane is so fucking basic anyway.

Showing this side of yourself takes balls to begin with. Much bigger balls than it takes to hide behind the full-time lad persona. But after a while it becomes easy-peasy. By doing it you're not only helping yourself – you are helping other blokes around you. I know this because having a mate like Dan is a gift and a privilege. By being honest about himself he gives me licence to be more honest about myself. And being more honest about myself is truly liberating.

What have you got to hide when you are completely upfront about yourself? Nothing. And if you're not hiding anything then you have less reason to be anxious. If you're less anxious then you're less likely to indulge in self-destructive behaviour.

It's not just Dan: I am lucky to have a number of mates who are just as honest, vulnerable and fun to be with. I've ditched the ones who aren't. Once you open yourself up to this stuff, you find it easy to shed those blokes for whom every social encounter is a tedious game of one-upmanship.

Being pissed in the pub all the time is all right – for kiddies. It's pretty boring and exhausting to put all that energy into pretending to be stronger than the next bloke. Constantly giving it the Big One is for babies, bullshitters and the sort of pompous, trumped-up arseholes who currently run the country. Leave all that Billy Big Bollocks stuff to the public school wankers and drippy golf-club bores.

Proper grown-ups, with a real pair of bollocks on them, go and look at the otters and talk about their insecurities. Talk to your mates. Ask them how they are. In turn, they will be more likely to check in on you when you're struggling. It's all about small steps. You don't have to suddenly start going to primal scream therapy in the woods. You're not going to become the Dalai Lama overnight. You don't need to be.

Saturday 25 June 2022 marked my seven-year sober anniversary. It's an occasion I like to mark, but not one I celebrate. I don't feel particularly proud of it. I still feel ashamed that I allowed my drinking and drug taking to get so out of hand. But I am also strangely grateful because, through the experience of addiction and recovery, I discovered a new way of living that is so much more pleasant.

That Saturday I put up a shelf in our utility room. Then I went to football training with my son. In the evening, we had a takeaway and watched *Kenobi* on Disney Plus. Just my wife, my daughter, my son and me, all slumped together on the sofas, eating, laughing, taking the piss out of each other. I try not to overthink those moments but, on Saturday, I did take a breath and reflected a little bit on how safe and relaxed and surrounded by love I felt. I didn't feel proud. I felt lucky and grateful.

I put a picture of myself on social media announcing that I was seven years sober. I talk publicly about it because I want people who are in the same situation that I was once in to see that there is a way out. I was a fucking mess back in 2015. I thought things had gone so far that I might drop dead. Losing my wife, my kids and my career had started to seem possible – maybe even probable. I had lost all faith in myself. I just didn't think I would ever find a way out of the bad habits that had come to define my existence.

But I did. And now I've got a happy and calm life that is defined by love, not fear. I'm not sure I am capable of showing anyone the way out of their own private hell. All I can do is show them that I did it, so they can too.

That's the message I want you to take from this book. I've tried not to glorify my drunken antics. There is a tendency among recovering addicts to relive the old days as if they are something cool and glamorous.

But it's all bollocks. There was nothing cool or funny about my drinking and drug taking. Yes, when I was younger I had some good times. But I fooled myself into thinking that I had control. The problems crept up on me sneakily as I got older. There wasn't a single trigger. Drinking and taking drugs had just become too normalised for me over the years, so eventually they were able to take control of my life without me even noticing.

When it got bad, in those last couple of years, it was boring and lonely and weird and depressing. It wasn't like being a member of Fleetwood Mac in the 1970s. I was on my own in the living room late at night, creeping around while my family slept upstairs. I was in the corner of the pub at lunchtime, downing whisky chasers and endless pints between lines of coke in the stinking toilet. I was slipping vodka into my orange juice to hide my boozing from my wife. I was doing coke at work to prepare for meetings. It was an endless cycle of inebriation followed by hangovers followed by more inebriation to stave off the demons of misery and fear that followed me like vultures.

I was just so fucking sad all the time. I felt trapped and unable to re-engage with the positive, happy, honest parts of my life because I'd allowed booze and drugs to drag me away from them. I felt like I couldn't tell anyone about it. I was ashamed of my bad habits so I kept them secret. I felt alone and isolated and too scared to open up and ask for help.

Nowadays, when I talk about this stuff, people say things like: 'I had no idea you had such a big problem.' That's because I was working overtime to hide everything about myself. I was scared that I would be judged or rejected or condemned. The lying and dishonesty only increased the sense of shame and self-hatred, which, in turn, increased my desire to numb my feelings with booze and drugs. It was a vicious circle. But when I eventually found the courage to tell the truth about what was happening to me, I was delighted to discover that people reacted with sympathy and love. The people who mattered, anyway. The others, I just had to distance myself from.

A few people congratulated me on my willpower. But the truth is that my sobriety requires no willpower at all. I fucking hated every minute of being a pissed-up cokehead. There are no happy memories, just awful ones. The thought of having drink or drugs ever again is absolutely abhorrent to me.

Everything good in my life is based on a foundation of sobriety. I wouldn't have my wife or my kids or a career that I love if I wasn't sober. Staying this way is not a chore. It's not hard work. It's easy to be sober. What's hard is being someone who can't remember how to function without drugs and drink inside them. The hardest thing I have to cope with nowadays is wrestling with the feelings of guilt and shame that still sometimes haunt me; reminders of the stupid habits into which I once let myself fall. But I'm getting better at staving off those thoughts.

You might not have a problem with booze or drugs. But everyone goes through bad times of anxiety, depression, self-doubt and discomfort. Even those of us who seem to have it made. I am so glad that my addictions drove me to sort my head out. I hope you can sort yours out without having to reach such a state of desperation first. Remember, you can't be the great dad, husband, boyfriend, son, brother or friend you want to be unless you're taking care of yourself first and foremost. Sort your own head out before you try to sort out anything else.

If you're struggling, show yourself a little love. Try not to beat yourself up about your situation. Recognise when you are in a bad place and that you need a bit of kindness and love to navigate your way out of it. With any luck, you will get that from the people around you. But you can start by giving it to yourself.

Help and Acknowledgements

Some services, links and phone numbers to help you through the tough times:

www.samaritans.org; tel. 116 123
@thecalmzone; tel. 0800 58 58 58
@YoungMindsUK; tel. 0800 018 2138
@CharitySane; tel. 0300 304 7000
www.alcoholics-anonymous.org.uk
www.cocaineanonymous.org.uk
andysmanclub.co.uk
www.nhs.uk/live-well/healthy-body/gambling-addiction/
samdelaney.substack.com

There are two sets of people who made this book possible. First, I'd like to thank those who actually helped the publishing process: Andreas Campomar at Constable for believing in the project from the start and supporting me with such passion. Also, Holly Blood at Constable for her warm, wise and diligent editorial guidance. And Howard Watson for his shrewd, thorough and very helpful copyedit. And my agent Matthew Hamilton for all of his support and friendship over the years.

re are the people who helped me get through all of
l downs described in this book. Many of you might
how important you have been to me and what a
positive role you have played in my life.

First, all the lads I grew up with, with special mention to Hack, an excellent mate through thick and thin.

There are people who have inspired me along the way with their own courage, love and intelligence: Dan Foley and Alice Sinton foremost among them.

There have been friends and colleagues who got me through some of the toughest moments of my life by being loyal and compassionate: not least my pod husband, friend and 'rock' Mr Andy Dawson. Phil Hilton has been a brilliant friend and mentor throughout my career and offered wise counsel on the title and cover of this book. I am grateful to him, always.

Also, Mark Machado and Jay Pond-Jones, thank you.

I am also grateful to everyone who has supported *The Reset* over the past few years. Whether you subscribed or appeared on the podcast, thanks so much for making all this happen. I am grateful to my mate Anna Stewart for encouraging me to write and talk about this stuff publicly. Also thanks to Kay Ribeiro for being one of the first to suggest I should write this book and championing the whole project.

Massive thanks to the professionals who have helped me grow into a better person over the past seven years: Dr Niall Campbell, Jordan Griffiths and, of course, the magnificent Lizann.

I am grateful, always, to my mum and dad. Love you both.

To Annie, thanks for being the best big sister in the world.

To MJ, thanks for being the best little sister in the world.

Coco and Len – I am so proud of you both and love you more than anything. Thanks for making life so brilliant.

Anna, you are the love of my life and I wouldn't have been able to do any of this without you. Thanks for everything, always.